MW00959445

Glucose Revolution Hacks

Unlocking the Secrets to Healthy Glucose Levels for Optimal Health, Prime Wellness, and Longevity

Olivia Rivers

© Copyright 2023 - All rights reserved.

The content contained within this book may not be reproduced, duplicated or transmitted without direct written permission from the author or the publisher.

Under no circumstances will any blame or legal responsibility be held against the publisher, or author, for any damages, reparation, or monetary loss due to the information contained within this book, either directly or indirectly.

Legal Notice:

This book is copyright protected. It is only for personal use. You cannot amend, distribute, sell, use, quote or paraphrase any part, or the content within this book, without the consent of the author or publisher.

Disclaimer Notice:

Please note the information contained within this document is for educational and entertainment purposes only. All effort has been executed to present accurate, up to date, reliable, complete information. No warranties of any kind are declared or implied. Readers acknowledge that the author is not engaged in the rendering of legal, financial, medical or professional advice. The content within this book has been derived from various sources. Please consult a licensed professional before attempting any techniques outlined in this book.

By reading this document, the reader agrees that under no circumstances is the author responsible for any losses, direct or indirect, that are incurred as a result of the use of the information contained within this document, including, but not limited to, errors, omissions, or inaccuracies.

Your Exclusive Gift: 7-Day

Meal Plan for Glucose Success!

Are you ready to kickstart your journey towards optimal health and vitality? As a special gift to you, here is an exclusive 7-day meal plan designed to support you in mastering your glucose levels and achieving greater wellness.

Simply scan the QR code provided, and get ready to embark on a delicious and transformative culinary adventure that will fuel your success on the path to balanced glucose and vibrant well-being.

Here's to your health, success, and a revolutionary glucose journey ahead!

Table of Contents

Introduction

If you live in the modern world, then you live under a constant barrage of diet advice. By now, if you are in your 40s, you have lived through Atkins (which is coming back), keto, the Zone diet, and, if you remember, the South Beach Diet. Your web browser throws ads at you saying things like, "Doctors Are Literally BEGGING People To Stop Eating This One Food!" And, of course, celebrities are constantly backing this or that trick to get slim quick.

Interestingly enough, however, this is nothing new and not limited to this period in history. As far back as ancient Rome, people were taking part in fad diets, some of which involved eating large amounts of deer liver. Lord Byron, the great English poet, was an ardent follower of fad diets.

In some ways, it feels like we are on a treadmill we will never get off of. One thing follows another, which gets discarded when another comes along. Forever and ever.

What we need, then, is a diet which is backed by nutritional science. One which has the facts to back it up. One which can deliver on its promises.

Enter: the glucose revolution.

As it turns out, glucose—or "blood sugar," as it is commonly known—is not just something diabetics should be concerned with. Glucose, and in particular the level of glucose in our blood, is associated with all kinds of health effects. And learning to control our levels of glucose is going to open up those effects for us in ways we can only imagine.

For me, this wasn't an easy lesson to learn. But I can trace its genesis all the way back to something that happened when I was only a teenager. And it has informed my attitude on this ever since.

I was in the sixth grade and was out on a field trip. There was an emu farm out in the rural area outside where I lived, and we were to spend the day there. The idea was we would learn not just about emus, but about large, flightless birds at the little museum they had.

We left on the bus first thing in the morning. I sat somewhere in the middle, next to the new girl, Shana Rey. She had just moved from out of state and was having trouble making friends because she was so shy. I thought she seemed nice, so I sat with her.

Not far from school, I noticed Shana pull out a bag of blueberries. It was a little plastic bag but it was filled with fruits, which she kept in the breast pocket of her shirt. When she took out a handful, I found myself getting hungry and asked if I could have some.

She held them tight to her chest and shook her head.

"You can't," she said. "I need them."

"What do you mean you need them?"

"I'm diabetic. I have to keep my blood sugar level."

I did not know what that meant at the time. But still, I did not feel like I should pry. It felt like something very personal, that she would not want to share with others.

When we got to the emu farm, we filed out of the bus slowly and single file. It was a hot day, and the open country made the sun seem that much hotter. Shana, I remember, was already sweating by the time we walked off the bus stairs and onto the hard dirt.

To this day, I do not know if maybe being sweaty was what did it. She was holding onto the railing that led down the bus stairs and maybe her hand slipped. Maybe there was something on the stairs themselves, I do not know.

What I do know is she tripped and fell. And landed right on the blueberries.

There was a bit of a commotion after that, I remember. Shana was scared about her diabetes. The teachers seemed to be also, but they assured her there would be plenty to eat when lunch came around and that so long as she ate breakfast, she should be fine.

It was on the way to the emu pen that Shana turned to me and said, "I skipped breakfast."

"You did what?" I said. "Why didn't you tell them?"

"I don't wanna be trouble." She looked worried. "I'm gonna be okay, right?"

I said she would. But I knew nothing about diabetes. The truth was, I had no idea.

And boy, was I ever wrong.

It happened when I first fed one of the emus. If you have never seen one, they are pretty amazing creatures. Tall, with crazy eyes. And when they open their mouths, there is a black hole in their throats that seems to go on forever.

I had some feed in my hand, which I threw into the pen. One of the big emus was in front of me and he ate what I had thrown in there. I was absorbed in this creature, watching him move. It was like looking at an alien.

But that moment lasted only a second. Because from behind me, I heard someone scream.

I can say now that what happened was due to hypoglycemia. At the time, however, I had no idea what was going on. All I knew was that the new girl was on her back, her eyes had rolled into the back of her head and someone, one of the teachers, was jabbing a needle into her side.

It was a horrifying moment. I was totally frozen, more like a scarecrow than a young girl. I really thought I was going to see someone die.

Thankfully, Shana lived. She did not last much longer at our school, because her dad was in the air force, and they had to move a lot. And in truth, I have no idea what happened to her after that.

But seeing that was a watershed moment for me. Because I wanted to make sense of what I had seen. I asked the adults and teachers in my life to explain it to me and I heard words like "diabetes," which I already knew from Shana, and "blood sugar" and all the rest. But I wanted—really wanted—to know how something so strange and mind-numbing had happened to Shana.

And what I learned in the years since only convinced me more so about how important glucose is.

So, yes, I can trace my interest in glucose back to that moment. And everything I have learned about it, I have tried to put into this book.

Throughout this book, we are going to learn about what glucose is and how it affects us. We are going to learn all about how our body regulates it and what we can do to manage that. We are going to talk about food, both what we eat and how we eat it.

And we are going to use this to unlock a whole host of benefits, from sleep and mental well-being, all the way up to longevity.

I can't promise you this is going to be easy. But I can promise you that it is going to be simple. Because really, in many cases, our health essentially comes down to blood sugar.

So, with that said, let's strap in. Because we have lots of ground to cover. But in the end, everything we cover is only going to keep us healthy, happy, and help to ensure that we live a long life.

It is time to join the glucose revolution.

Chapter 1:

Understanding Glucose and Its

Role in The Body

Dylan Thomas opened *Under Milk Wood* with the line, "To begin at the beginning." This is probably one of the most recognizable first lines in history, right after "Call me Ishmael." It is probably because, as with anything, there is never a better place to start than with where a thing begins.

For us, the beginning is going to be some definitions. Before we get to the nitty-gritty, we need to know what exactly the thing is that we are dealing with.

Which means we will need to start by asking: Just what is glucose?

Discover the Hidden Secrets of Glucose: Why It Matters More Than You Think!

We hear a lot of talk about "carbs," or "carbohydrates," if you are not into the whole brevity thing. Nonetheless, many of us will not know that a carb is one of the sources our body uses for fuel; this, along with fat and protein. We also might not know that if carbs are a species, then glucose is the genus—in other words, glucose is a type of carb, in fact, the simplest type (Wright & Dias, 2022).

Going a little further here, glucose is what we would call a "monosaccharide," which is a fancy word meaning "one sugar." There are other types of monosaccharide, including fructose, galactose, and ribose. These forms of dietary glucose and carbs are converted by the body into blood sugar, which gives us energy (Wright & Dias, 2022).

Now, a carb is either simple or complex, and is called as such because of how quickly the sugar is digested. That is another thing we hear a lot about—simple and complex carbs. Simple carbs are things like pasta, table sugar and soda. Complex carbs include things like brown rice, oats, and fruit (Wright & Dias, 2022).

One thing we might tell by looking at those examples is that complex carbs are considered healthier choices than simple ones. Why is this? Well, complex carbs take longer to break down in the body, which gives us energy for longer. The simple ones are a cause of our glucose levels dipping and spiking rapidly, which can have undesirable effects on our health (Wright & Dias, 2022).

"But hold on," you might say. "This is all fine and good, but I think you are overlooking the role the pancreas plays in all this!"

Just kidding, I know you are not saying that. But in case you are, you would be right. And so with that in mind, we should turn to the pancreas and its effect on our blood sugar levels.

Your body begins breaking down what you eat almost immediately. Specifically, your body is looking to get a hold of glucose and other carbohydrates with the help of the pancreas. This organ produces many hormones, but insulin is the one we are interested in right now, since it is essential to managing the rise in blood sugar you get from eating (Wright & Dias, 2022).

So yes, ye lover of all things pancreas, that organ plays a crucial role in our health. But specifically, for our purpose, we are going to interest ourselves with the hormone insulin and the role that it plays in our well-being. And more specifically, what we know or can learn about diabetes, and how we can extrapolate from that to other aspects of our health.

Diabetes, then, is what happens when the pancreas does not release insulin in the way it should. This is why diabetics need insulin injections, to help manage this (Wright & Dias, 2022).

But the other way in which diabetes occurs is from insulin resistance. Essentially, your cells do not recognize that insulin has been released, which results in too much blood sugar. This, in turn, begins a chain reaction which leads to your blood pH reaching dangerous levels, in addition to the release of ketones. This is how a person reaches ketoacidosis, which can possibly kill you (Wright & Dias, 2022).

In other words, in case you hadn't heard, diabetes is an undesirable, life-threatening condition which requires a high degree of concern, both medicinally and otherwise, in order to maintain the person's health.

One of the ways in which people with diabetes concern themselves with their well-being is by monitoring their glucose levels. A doctor might, for example, ask a person with diabetes to monitor their levels before and after meals, before and after exercise, or before bedtime. This is done via a blood test, which involves sticking one's fingertip with a needle, applying the blood to a strip and placing the strip in a meter designed to test blood sugar (Wright and Dias, 2022).

But while people with diabetes have to do this consistently, there are times when they should be more concerned with their blood sugar than others. Shockingly, one of those times is when you get a sunburn, because the pain causes your blood sugar to go up. But more commonly than that, anything from skipping meals to trying new medication can alter your blood sugar level to a concerning status and should be monitored closely.

What this means essentially, is that blood sugar is an integral part of our well-being. When our bodies' regulatory mechanisms regarding glucose get out of whack, things get hairy, and we wind up having to take extra steps to keep that on track.

So far so good. But with that in mind, let's take a deeper dive into how our body regulates blood sugar.

Cracking the Code: Understanding How Your Body Regulates Glucose

Do we know what the word "autonomically" means?

In case you do not, it means "involuntarily." I know, a weird way to start off. But it is not just an important word, it is an important concept—at least for us, right now.

Why, you ask? Well, one of the things about how our body regulates glucose, and which should, frankly, be obvious, is that the whole process is done autonomically. And not only that, but it's done constantly, too (Long, 2020).

Effectively, we have no control over this process. Certainly, we are required to eat what is healthy for us and shun what is not, and refusing to do so can harm our blood sugar levels. But the actual process of breaking it down is done without any conscious input from us whatsoever.

As we discussed earlier, the pancreas is what regulates our blood sugar levels, and it does this through the release of various hormones. These are insulin, which lowers your blood glucose (BG) levels; glucagon, which elevates it; and somatostatin, which regulates between the two, essentially by turning each one off and on (Long, 2020).

This is how the whole thing works: You eat food which contains carbs, which is then digested, causing BG levels to rise. The pancreas responds with insulin, shutting off glucagon production. This is in an effort to balance your BG levels out. The glucose that is in your blood then enters the liver, which starts a reaction that ends in a series of enzymes converting glucose in glycogen

This is where you enter what is called a "postprandial state," which is a fancy way of saying you have been "fed." During this state, the liver is taking in more glucose than it is releasing. Eventually, your BG levels drop from having digested all that food, which is when your insulin production drops. The liver then has all this fancy glucose it can release when the body needs energy (Long, 2020).

If this is interesting to you, then great! There are so many other resources you can explore, from books to videos, to everything in between, which can expand your knowledge about this subject.

In fact, I encourage you to do it. Getting to know how our bodies work will only encourage us to be healthier!

But now that we have a decent base from which to jump, we need to get into some of the more pressing matters. Like, for instance, what happens when our glucose levels get all out of whack.

"Unveiling the Silent Threat: The Dangers of Imbalanced Glucose Levels"

As I am sure you know, the state of having low blood sugar is called hypoglycemia, while the state of having high blood sugar is called hyperglycemia. Neither of these is desirable, but each of them has its own set of complications associated with it.

With that in mind—let's take a dive into both!

Starting with hyperglycemia: As stated above, this is when you have too much blood sugar, or, put another way, your blood glucose levels are too high. If this has happened to you, it probably means your body is not producing insulin, or that you have developed insulin resistance (Cleveland Clinic, 2020).

Having hyperglycemia also likely means you have diabetes. And if you do have hyperglycemia but refuse to treat it for long periods of time, well, are you ever in trouble! Cleveland Clinic has some helpful information to offer about this condition (2020).

Over the long term, the condition will likely damage your nerves, cells and organs. It can also lead to a life-threatening form of ketoacidosis specific to diabetics. Even in the short term, you can expect everything from frequent urination, increased thirst or hunger, and blurred vision. In the long term, you can also look forward to sores, wounds that will not heal quickly, vaginal yeast infections, and fatigue.

The diabetic ketoacidosis is not a walk in the park either. You will wind up with nausea and vomiting, fruity-smelling breath, dehydration, abdominal pain, difficulty breathing, increased heart rate, and confusion. All of these, by the way, are the kinds of symptoms over which you will want to call a doctor.

As stated earlier, hyperglycemia can be caused by insulin resistance, which is what happens when your body, specifically the cells in your muscles, fat and liver, is not responding to insulin in the way that it should. This makes your pancreas produce more insulin, but when it cannot produce enough, you wind up with hyperglycemia.

This, by the way, is the main cause of type 2 diabetes. But this form of diabetes can also be caused by obesity, especially when the kind of fat you have is centered in your abdomen; physical inactivity; a diet that is high in sugary processed junk; and certain types of medication, which can include some treatments for HIV and various psychiatric drugs.

Also—we should not forget about hormonal problems, because those are key too. This can include problems with growth hormone or cortisol (stress hormone). It is because of this that pregnancy too can lead to what is known as gestational diabetes, which is not a fun condition to have either.

And what about damage to the pancreas? Can this have an effect on your blood sugar, also?

Why, yes it can! Type 1 diabetes, for example, is an autoimmune disease in which your immune system attacks your pancreas, for reasons that remain a mystery. Once this happens, your insulin production goes haywire, causing diabetes. Prolonged inflammation of the pancreas too (commonly known as pancreatitis) can lead to hyperglycemia, as can pancreatic cancer and cystic fibrosis.

And what are some of the complications which arise from chronic, untreated hyperglycemia? Well, how about retinopathy, which is when the blood vessels in your eyes become weak, causing vision loss and, yes, blindness? Or, if you prefer, there is always nephropathy, which is a disease affecting your kidneys;

this is what causes the excessive urination in diabetics and, yes, the foamy pee.

We have all heard of cases of people who lose their feet to diabetes. This is because of neuropathy, which is where diabetes affects the nerve cells, specifically in the extremities. There is also gastroparesis, which is when your stomach becomes paralyzed, causing food to sit in it for dangerous amounts of time.

And finally, we have two heavy hitters: heart disease and stroke.

In summary, a motley crew, a veritable rogues' gallery of horrible things that can happen to you, all because of prolonged, elevated blood sugar levels. Ensuring, therefore, that these levels do not get too high for too long, is not just an important aspect of a healthy lifestyle, it is, judging by the complications associated with it, maybe one of the top ones.

Hypoglycemia, its opposite, is no walk in the park either. It has numerous causes, including the amount of physical activity you do, drinking too much alcohol, the amount of fat, protein and fiber in your diet, hot and humid weather, and spending too much time at high altitudes (Center for Disease Control and Prevention (CDC), 2021). In essence, if you are the drunk hockey player in Aspen during the summertime with a poor diet, you are probably hypoglycemic.

How do you know if you have low blood sugar? Well, many of us will have experienced bouts of this at some point or another. So, we will be familiar with the elevated heart rate, shaking, and sweating. But there are also instances of people feeling nervous or anxious, confused, and dizzy.

However, if you have been dealing with low blood sugar for five-to-ten years, there is a good chance you might not have any symptoms at all. This adds an extra challenge into the mix, namely that if you do not notice any symptoms, you will not know that your blood sugar has dropped and will not, therefore, treat the problem.

There are different types of low blood sugar too. One of these is called nighttime low blood sugar, which can be especially hairy given that you are almost certainly asleep when it happens. This can be caused by getting drunk before bed, taking too much insulin, or being active close to bedtime (CDC, 2021).

This can be prevented a number of different ways, but if you do drink alcohol before bed, it is advisable to also eat. While you might wake up when your blood sugar drops, the only way to really be sure of it is to have a glucose monitor on you while you are sleeping (CDC, 2021).

Severe episodes of low blood sugar, meanwhile, comes with a whole host of symptoms, none of which are desirable in the slightest. For example, you can become weak, have difficulty walking or seeing clearly, acting "strange," becoming confused, and God help us, having seizures.

Needless to say, this is a horrible state of affairs which will require medical intervention. If you think you might be at risk of low blood sugar, therefore, you will want to get a snack in before letting the problem become so severe that you have a seizure.

Which leaves us where, exactly? Well, as we have seen, there is an absolute, direct link between our blood sugar levels and our wellbeing. Like the Goldilocks story, there is too much, there is too little, and there is just right. And we, of course, want just right.

But as we go on here, we are going to realize that this really is only half the picture. Monitoring our blood sugar is not just about making sure we do not have seizures, or preventing episodes of confusion, elevated heart rate, and chronic tissue damage.

These things are all great. But there is more to the story than just that.

Fuel Up for Success: Unlocking the Power of Optimal Glucose Levels

Part of the problem with what we might call "high glucose variability," or glucose levels that are going way far up and way far down, and doing so frequently, is that your body has to work extra hard to try and keep those levels stable. This can be part of what brings on insulin resistance (Johnson, 2022).

(It should be noted, however, that there is reason to think that insulin resistance is associated more with fat than it is with glucose. But for our purposes, we can put that aside, if only for the time being).

Reversing insulin resistance is only going to help us. Think of all the diseases you can reverse or avoid altogether: prediabetes, obesity, type 2 diabetes. Additionally, it may also help with things like fatigue and inflammation (Johnson, 2022).

All of which is worth thinking about. But that is by no means the whole picture. In fact, as we will soon see, there are a whole bunch of other reasons why we should be interested in monitoring our glucose.

One of the things we might not associate with glucose regulation, is what we would call "healthspan." Whereas "lifespan" refers to the amount of time you live for, "healthspan" refers to how much of your life is spent in good health (Johnson, 2022).

This should be clear when we think of all the ailments associated with poor glucose production. Obesity, for example, is an indicator of poor health. But other metabolic-related illnesses, like insulin resistance, are also predictors of various age-related health problems. These include such illustrious characters as cancer, heart disease and stroke

Additionally, there is some research which suggests that there may be a link between insulin resistance and brain health. "Brain health" here refers to issues like cognitive decline, as well as other brain-related pathologies. This happens because of how diabetes affects neurons, essentially by creating signaling problems which lead to issues like cognitive decline (Johnson, 2022).

And how about this: Insulin resistance and waist circumference are associated with the shortening of blood cell chromosomes, which is what happens as you age (Johnson, 2022). In essence, insulin resistance is aging you faster than your normal rate.

So, yes, it is possible that by regulating your glucose levels, and not developing insulin resistance, you might increase the total amount of time in your life that you spend in good health. Not bad!

Another thing we should know about too, is that blood glucose affects our endocrine system, which is what produces hormones.

This, by the way, includes some of the heavy hitters, like stress and sex hormones, as well as those that regulate our appetites (Johnson, 2022).

So, yes, not managing your glucose can have an effect on your sex life. Need I say more?

But also, decreased levels of estrogen in women might heighten the risk of cancer. Specifically, cancers of the ovaries and breast (Johnson, 2022). Which means that, while hormones are most often linked with behavior and mood and things like that, hormone dysfunction can have far-reaching, medically interesting effects on other, vital areas of our lives.

Take, for example, the link between glucose and cortisol. High glucose is associated with an increase in cortisol, which is a stress hormone. If cortisol levels remain high for long periods of time, all sorts of rotten things follow. These commonly include inflammation and weight gain, for starters (Johnson, 2022). But high cortisol levels are also associated with cancer, as if weight gain wasn't bad enough on its own.

And speaking of weight gain!

If your glucose level has lots of, and frequent, high peaks and low valleys, and a fasting glucose that is abnormally high (meaning your base level glucose without introducing food), then you can not only gain weight, but have a harder time getting rid of it.

Essentially what happens, according to some research, is that fatty tissue makes insulin signaling more difficult. But in addition to that, overweight and obese people are at greater risk for insulin sensitivity (Johnson, 2022).

The way to fix this, obviously, is to make better food choices, exercise—we know the drill. But obviously, given the gamut of things that you become at risk for when you let your glucose levels go haywire, this is something we should be desirous to fix.

Which begs the question: Is that all we are really talking about doing here? Staving off cancer and weight gain? Are there no out right positives to monitoring our glucose levels?

I mean, first off, if that was your question, then your outlook is in need of a tune-up. But additionally, yes, there are outright positives to monitoring your glucose levels. And we are going to go through some of them here!

How about this to kick things off: Your energy levels can be better managed.

When you eat a meal high in refined carbs, your blood glucose becomes elevated. This not only makes you feel tired, but gives you brain fog (Johnson, 2022). Eating complex carbs will give you the energy needed to last the day, which means, yes, avoiding the ol' afternoon slump.

And what about improvements in your mood? Well, some research has linked high glucose variability to irritability and anxiety. So for those of us who are stressed out a good chunk of the time, it might be that we need to consider our diet as a possible culprit. Changing that might actually make us feel better and less prone to anger (Johnson, 2022).

That still not good enough for you? Alright then, what about the fact that you will experience fewer food cravings? Yes, you heard that right. Because as it turns out, some of our cravings for sweet foods come from our blood sugar spiking from refined sugars, only to crash dramatically soon after. Our body knows we need sugar to make up for the crash, so we crave those sugary treats that are oh, so bad for us (Johnson, 2022).

Do you have cravings for food like that on an alarming basis? Do you think that might be part of the reason why you are having trouble losing weight? Consider this as a possibility then!

And finally, yes, it is possible that balancing your glucose levels might give you better skin. This is kind of a complicated one, but remember how our glycemic diet affects sex hormones? Well, it turns out that our sex hormones also affect our skin health. Essentially, when we have a high glycemic diet, our sex hormones start a process of production that leads to oily skin. Oily skin, as we know, is a cause of breakouts (Johnson, 2022).

As teenagers, many of us had to deal with the dreaded acne breakouts. It was all a part of the David Cronenberg nightmare that is puberty. Our bodies changed in ways that, for many of us, felt like becoming a human fly.

Okay, that might be an exaggeration. But still! Having to go through the acne problem as a teenager is bad enough that we all hope being an adult means the end of that particular worry. If the worry has continued to dog us since our adolescence, is it possible that our diet is the culprit?

It just might be. And if so, then the solution is as simple as altering the kind of sugars we take in during our meals. (In addition to some other things, but for now that is not a bad start).

So where, then, does that leave us?

Well, we know a little about what glucose is now. We know about its role in the body, about diabetes, and about the pancreas' role in the whole thing. We also know what might happen to us risk-wise if we do not manage our blood sugar levels, and what benefits we might accrue from actually doing it.

I hope that this means we are on the same page. And that page says that our blood glucose is an integral part of our overall well being. And we would do well to monitor it and adopt healthy lifestyle choices to make sure it does not lead to negative health consequences.

But how do we do that?

In the coming chapter we will deal with some of the ways we can actually pull this off. We will get into food, sleep, exercise, the whole shebang.

I think I have pleaded my case sufficiently well, don't you?

Then let's get onto the good stuff. Let's talk about the tools we have at our disposal and get the process started on unlocking our wellbeing.

Chapter 2:

Factors Affecting Glucose

Levels

Now that we have an understanding of the basics—where do we go from here?

Well, as with anything, what you know is great, but knowing how to use it is even better. It is a lot like driving: You can read all the books you want, you can know cars inside and out, but if you want to be a good driver, you just have to buckle down and drive the damn thing.

Which is why, in this chapter, we are going to go through the specifics regarding what exactly affects our glucose levels. We are going to do this because we want to implement these changes into our lives so we can reap the benefits.

So, yes, my analogy was not exactly perfect. But whose is, am I right?

We are going to cover such fancy things as the glycemic index and how we can use that to better control our blood sugar. We are also going to look at exercise, which is, as always, one of the key ingredients to a healthy lifestyle.

But we are also going to look at maybe the most neglected aspect of our health: sleep. And we might even be surprised at what effect that has on our blood sugar!

With that said, let's dive in and learn about the glycemic index!

Food as Fuel: Navigating the Dietary Maze for Optimal Glucose Control

Who's heard of the glycemic index? Raise your hand.

Okay, I obviously can't see anybody's hands. But if I had to guess, I would think that while some of you had heard of this, most of you would not have. And of those of you with your hands raised, I would bet that most could not explain to me exactly what it is.

Which is fine! Because I am here, after all, to explain this. And I think it is an important one, which is why it is too bad that it is not talked about more.

To start then, the glycemic index is a categorization tool which defines just how much a certain food affects our blood sugar levels. We arrive at this number via various factors, such as nutrient composition and ripeness, but also how much process the food has undergone.

Essentially how it works is that the lower the GI rating, the less it affects your blood sugar. Low GI is defined as 55 or less, medium as 56-69, and high is 70+. A food with a high GI is probably processed and sugary, while foods with lots of protein and fiber most likely have a low GI (Ajmera, 2023).

So already we can see the positive effects this system can have. It allows us to spot foods that are most often junk, and to choose food that is healthier for us. White bread, with its high GI, is junk; apples, with their low GI, are the opposite of junk.

Additionally, foods without carbs are not assigned a GI. So all the meats, including fish, as well as herbs and spices, are not a part of this conversation, although their importance in a healthy diet will be. Which means, yes, that choosing healthy foods outside of the glycemic index is still important.

But within the foods we are talking about here—what are the benefits to choosing foods with a low GI?

Much of the research shows that doing so contributes to improved blood sugar regulation. For people with type 2 diabetes in particular, this is going to help ameliorate their condition. But even for those of us without T2D, doing this will only boost our overall health (Ajmera, 2023).

Perhaps even more obviously than that, there is a connection between eating low-GI foods and weight loss, specifically in the short term. Whether this continues in the long term is still not completely understood, but if short term weight loss is the goal, then this might be a sensible method to accomplish that.

And how about this—it looks like low-GI foods will help with fatty liver disease. However, and this is crucial, low-GI foods do not help with fatty liver as a result of alcohol misuse. Which is unfortunate, but such is the way of things.

So much for the benefits. Which foods should we be eating then to actually pull this off? Rachael Ajmera, MS, RD, of Healthline, explains this perfectly. The following advice takes inspiration from her article (Ajmera, 2023).

Fruits, of course. The noble fruit has come under fire in the last decade or so by Atkins and keto supporters. But do not listen to them! Fruit is great and great for you. They are healthy, they are tasty, and you can put them in all kinds of things. Some people, for example, might balk at the idea of putting them in salad, but those people are wrong. Fruits are excellent in salad.

"Nature's candy," indeed.

Some fruits you can enjoy on a low-GI diet include: apples, berries, oranges, lemons and grapefruit. Having apples around to snack on is always a great idea. But I have always had blueberries out to take by the handful, as well as to throw in, yes, salads, but also yogurt in the morning.

Non-starchy vegetables are on this list also. The poor potato is going to get short shrift here, but there are plenty of other vegetables that we can use in its place. This would include broccoli, carrots, and spinach. And since we are all adults now— i.e., not babies who make gross-out faces at the thought of eating broccoli—this is fantastic news.

For whole grains, you have such illustrious foods as quinoa (which is underrated), barley and oats. And of course you have legumes, including lentils and kidney beans. Even if we did not have any other foods on our list, that is not bad on its own. In fact, you could live like a king on all that.

But of course, there are foods which are not on the glycemic index but are still "permitted"—although, to pause here for a second, nothing about the glycemic index should imply that certain foods should be banned from your eating habits. We are all human and we all enjoy a good snack every now and again. Thinking about food in terms of what is "permitted" is only going to drive us crazy, lead to us not hitting our goals and, in the worst case scenario, developing an eating disorder.

So let that kind of thinking be anathema to you.

Anyway, we were talking about foods not on the glycemic index which are nonetheless a part of a healthy diet. Which would these include?

Meat is, of course, a staple in the human diet. Although in Western countries we tend to eat too much of it in comparison with other foods, meat is still important and should not be disregarded without having a plan in place to make up for its absence. (Taking B12 would be an example of this.)

So here, we can enjoy beef, lamb, bison, and pork. But also seafood, including tuna, salmon, shrimp and sardines; and poultry, which includes duck, chicken, goose and turkey.

Myself, I have enjoyed crocodile recently. I have no idea where it is in this conversation, but for those of you who are adventurous in your eating habits, I recommend giving it a try.

Moving on: Oils, such as olive oil, is of course a part of a healthy diet. But we should not forget about nuts, such as peanuts, almonds, and pistachios; nor seeds, herbs, and spices. Some whole grains too are integral and should not be eliminated.

But which foods should we consider leaving out of our diets?

Alas, many bread products tend to be high on the GI. This includes white bread, naan, pita bread, and a whole host of other things. Rice, too, including white and jasmine rice, tends to spike your blood sugar, which means you might want to say goodbye to them also. Alternatives abound, obviously, but it is not a bad idea to think about leaving these in the dust.

Cereals too have foods that are high on the ol' GI. We might remember the Seinfeld bit about how sugary cereals were when he was a boy? Well, that stands true today. Just look at foods like Count Chocula. Is there any reason we would think that is a healthy way to start our morning?

Unfortunately, instant oats are going to be included in this list too. I say "unfortunately," because I happen to love instant oats. But sacrifices must be made, and no less for me than the reader.

Still, starchy vegetables are the most unfortunate casualty here. Potatoes have a whole host of health benefits, but they are high on the glycemic index. Which sucks! But remember that this includes french fries also, and nobody in their right mind would claim that french fries are a part of a healthy diet.

Perhaps as an occasional treat, but the french fry is a commonly cited culprit when it comes to weight gain. So, yes, alas, the french fry is going to be sacrificed.

Other, more obvious ones include baked goods like doughnuts and pies; snacks, like chips and candy bars; and of course, sugary beverages like soda and juice. These ones really should require little explanation, but suffice it to say that even if we are not on a glucose diet, these kinds of foods, especially soda, should be avoided like the Plague.

As far as where specific foods fall on the glycemic index, I have found a handy-dandy list so we can start to think about composing a diet plan.

This is the list in full (Ajmera, 2023):

Vegetables:

- Carrots (boiled): 39

- Plantains (boiled): 66

- Sweet potatoes (boiled): 63

- Pumpkin (boiled): 74

- Potatoes (boiled): 78

Fruit:

- Apples: 36

- Strawberries: 41

- Dates: 42

- Oranges: 43

- Banana: 51

- Mango: 51

- Blueberries: 53

- Pineapple: 59

- Watermelon: 76

Sweeteners:

- Fructose: 15

- Coconut sugar: 54

- Maple syrup: 54

- Honey: 61

- Table sugar: 65

Grains:

- Barley: 28

- Quinoa: 53

- Rolled oats: 55

- Couscous: 65

- Popcorn: 65

- Brown rice: 68

- White rice: 73

- Whole wheat bread: 74

- White bread: 75

Dairy products and dairy alternatives:
- Soymilk: 34

- Skim milk: 37

- Whole milk: 39

- Ice cream: 51

- Rice milk: 86

Legumes:
- Soybeans: 16

- Kidney beans: 24

- Chickpeas: 28

- Lentils: 32

So, yes, let me start off by saying "You're welcome." But let's take a look at some things we might notice about this, some things that might lead us into the next topic of discussion.

Why is it—you might be asking—that some foods I have listed here, are specifically listed as "boiled"? Does boiling them make some kind of a difference in its GI?

This will likely surprise you, but yes, how you cook some food does, in fact, change where it falls on the glycemic index.

For example, to start with a more obvious one, frying foods means increasing the amount of fat in the meal. Fat slows down the absorption of sugar, which would decrease the GI. But if you roast or bake foods, you wind up breaking down starch, which increases the GI. On the other hand, boiling might help food retain starch, which would decrease the GI.

When we cook foods like rice and pasta, one thing to keep in mind is that the longer we cook them, the more digestible they become. The more digestible they become, the higher their GI. Sort of a catch-22, considering that most of us don't like our rice to be anything other than soft.

But nonetheless, it is better for our blood sugar if we cook to reach an "al dente" texture, meaning that the pasta or rice are still firm. It is actually not as bad as it sounds, surprisingly enough. I have even come to prefer it! Especially knowing how much healthier it is.

And it is not just how we cook something that affects its GI either, but, if we are talking about fruit, a food's ripeness that does so.

Take bananas, for example. Bananas are starchy, especially when they are green. But notice how, as a banana ripens, it gets softer. This is because the banana is losing its starch through the ripening process. As this happens, the banana increases its GI.

The difference is fairly dramatic, also. A ripe banana has a GI of 51, whereas an underripe one has a GI of 30 (Ajmera, 2023). Like I said, huge difference.

In summary then: The glycemic index is a really, really useful tool. If we decide to go with the glucose diet as I am recommending in this book, then this is a fantastic way to monitor what our food is doing to our blood sugar levels.

And of course, as always, the amount of information out there is enormous. If you like what you have read in this chapter and want to know more, the internet or the library will be your friend. Look for books and articles on the glycemic index, learn as much as you possibly can, and decide for yourself if this is right for you.

In other words, since there is way more information out there than I can possibly put in this book, you can consider this chapter a pitch to get you interested in the subject. Hopefully it worked!

But, alas, it is time to move on. Because as much as we could talk about the glycemic index all day, we have to get into our next big topic: exercise.

Unlock The Power of Movement: How Physical Activity Transforms Glucose Health

We all know that exercise is one of the crucial elements to a healthy lifestyle. We know that it is an important part of heart and brain health; that putting on muscle helps maintain a high metabolism, and thereby allows us to burn more fat throughout the day.

We know all this. But do we know that exercise also helps with our blood sugar levels?

Well, if not, we are about to!

First things first: The relationship between exercise and blood glucose is nothing if not complicated. So, there will likely be some caveats along the way, along with some admissions of ambiguity.

For example, both of these statements are true: Exercise lowers your blood glucose; exercise raises your blood glucose. And in fact, understanding why this is so is one of the keys to unlocking the effect exercise has on our blood glucose (Collier, 2023).

See, when you exercise, your body is relying on either glucose or fat for energy, depending on the type of exercise you are doing. Your blood sugar is going to change, therefore, with regard to the type and intensity of the exercise you are doing (Collier, 2023).

"Steady-state exercises," for example, are those which do not rely on quick bursts of energy. Think here of jogging or swimming. Because of this, your body will get its energy from fat, which makes your blood sugar either stay at the same level, or else decrease (Collier, 2023).

Contrast this with what are known as HIIT workouts, or, "High intensity interval training." These involve things like strength training or sprinting, where your body releases adrenaline to accomplish its task. This is usually done, as you would expect, in intervals, where you give your body a rest and then go at it again, pushing yourself to work out in short, intense bursts.

In order to pull this kind of feat off, your liver releases glucose into your blood. This means, you guessed it, your blood sugar will spike while you are exercising. This is because your body does not have the energy in its resting state that is needed for high intensity training. In effect, the demand for energy goes up, so your body has to increase its supply.

And yet, despite these spikes in blood sugar in the short term, the long term effects of exercising on our blood sugar is positive. (In fact, these spikes are not in themselves negative; this is just how our body meets the energy demand!)

But how is this possible?

As we know now, when eating or resting, our body releases insulin when our blood sugar rises. This leads to our body storing glucose in the liver. But when we exercise, we increase the glucose uptake into our muscles, without having to use insulin

And what is more, this process can occur even in people with insulin resistance or diabetes. So, exercising for diabetics is an important part of managing the disease (Collier, 2023).

Another interesting thing exercise does relates to how it affects mitochondria. For those of you who have not taken biology in a long time (no judgment), mitochondria are the "powerhouse" of the cell; essentially, it is where the cell gets its energy. How this is done is by converting glucose into both oxygen, and a substance called adenosine triphosphate.

One thing that exercise appears to do is increase the number of mitochondria in your muscle cells. Which means that the more you exercise, the more of your muscles' glucose is turned into energy. Once this happens, you become more insulin sensitive. Which means, in summary, that you become less likely to develop diabetes (Collier, 2023).

Pretty cool, right?

And that is only the tip of the iceberg. Exercise also shrinks your fat cells, improves your ability to oxidize, or "burn fat," and clears your glycogen stores as it improves your ability to accumulate glycogen in the first place (Collier, 2023).

So yes, exercise is good for you. Who knew?

But which types of exercise are going to be best for our purposes?

Weight training is one of the key ingredients to any exercise regimen. This includes weight lifting (whether free or machine), all the different types of bodyweight exercises, and those cool resistance band workouts. The purpose of these exercises is to make you strong and increase your endurance.

Weight training is a type of exercise known as "anaerobic." This means that it uses glucose primarily, which is going to lead to improved blood sugar control and insulin sensitivity. In fact, for people with type 2 diabetes, strength training might even be preferable to cardio for managing the condition (Collier, 2023).

What happens when you engage in weight training, is that you gain lean muscle mass. Glycogen, again, is the space that stores glucose in your skeletal muscle and liver. This means that when you have more muscle, you have more space in which to store glucose.

Aerobic exercise, such as running, also has a positive effect on your blood glucose levels. This can be anything from jogging to swimming, at a consistent pace. And if you want to mix aerobic and anaerobic, then the HIIT workouts are really what you are looking for.

And do not forget about walking! It is such a simple exercise, but just walking at a reasonable pace is not only good for your overall health, but for your glucose levels specifically.

In summary then, while exercise does result in acute blood sugar spikes, the overall effect is that it evens your glucose levels out. Which means, yes, that exercise is still, next to food, the number one best thing you can possibly do for your health. Including for your blood sugar levels!

Which leaves us only with our final topic of the chapter: *sleep*.

From Stress to Serenity: How Sleep and Emotional Well-being Affect Our Blood Sugar

To begin with, much like exercise, sleep both increases and decreases your blood sugar levels. This has to do with our circadian rhythm—the cycle in which our body is naturally either asleep or awake. How this works is that your body increases blood sugar while you are sleeping, all on its own. Which means, yes, this is not something to worry about.

But poor sleep, especially a lack of sleep, can have a detrimental effect on our blood glucose. All it takes is one night of partial sleep deprivation to increase insulin resistance (Pacheco, 2020).

Which is wild, don't you think? This is, in fact, the reason sleep deprivation is linked to diabetes. So, making sure you are well-rested is going to have a preventive effect on your ability to become diabetic.

Now, it should be noted that there is still a lot more research that needs to be done. But for now, it looks as though the amount of time someone sleeps, the stages of sleep they experience, and the time of day they sleep, all impact blood sugar levels (Pacheco, 2020).

But why does this happen?

Okay, there are a few reasons. To begin with, as anyone who has been sleep deprived can testify, the experience is stressful. Cortisol, the stress hormone, is released when we do not get enough sleep, which increases glucose. Cortisol is also released depending on which time of day a person sleeps, while, additionally, inflammation is increased through sleep deprivation, which affects glucose.

There are other things too, such as our body releasing growth hormone at the same time as glucose when we sleep, and oxidative stress caused by sleep deprivation (Pacheco, 2020). All in all, poor sleep habits have a multifaceted effect on our bodies, which affects our hormones, which affect glucose.

But this also goes the other way, in that high blood sugar levels can make it harder for us to sleep. You can see how the vicious cycle begins here, where high blood sugar and poor sleep feed each other, making each one worse in turn.

Low blood sugar too has a whole host of problems associated with it. Some of these dreadful conditions include nightmares, yelling while asleep, sweating profusely, and being irritable or confused when you wake up. So, no matter which direction your blood sugar goes in, anything other than level is going to give you sleep problems.

In addition, there is a strong association between poor sleep patterns and sleep apnea. In fact, disordered breathing in general seems to be associated with high glucose levels, but this extends to everything from good old fashioned sleep apnea to the more extreme, obstructive sleep apnea (Pacheco, 2020).

Now, whether the sleep apnea is causing the glucose problems, or the other way around…? Hard to say. Obviously, given everything we have looked at here, one causes the other, which causes the other. The vicious cycle again.

Whichever winds up being the case, the connection between healthy sleep and healthy glucose seems, on its face, to be pretty rock solid, pending more research. So, getting one under control affects the other, and you wind up healthier as a result.

And in a society that is chronically sleep deprived, and chronically overweight, these conditions are very much worthy of our consideration.

But notice here that cortisol keeps coming up in the context of sleep deprivation. Stress, in other words, is one of the key influences on our well-being; especially since glucose and well-being are so closely intertwined with one another.

So, with that in mind, we should maybe take a quick detour into stress as a topic. We can investigate what kind of effect it can have on us in general, before dovetailing into how it affects glucose specifically.

First off, stress is a perfectly normal reaction to a whole host of life events. We all feel stressed when we have to start a new job, move, or, God forbid, when someone close to us dies. Money, of course, is a significant source of stress for people, and so financial instability is usually a good indicator of stress in a person.

When we get stressed, we have a whole host of symptoms that every single one of us is or will be familiar with. We get tense muscles, we get tired and grumpy, we have trouble staying asleep. These things happen.

When stress gets out of control, however, we start to get into dangerous territory. In a lot of cases, people will try to avoid the stressor at all costs. Often this means withdrawing from people, becoming isolated, or, in many cases, drinking or taking drugs more than usual.

For some people though, stress can be a positive thing. There are those among us who use stress as a sign of fuel, and can become more focused on this or that task at hand, under circumstances when they are stressed out.

If this is you, well, that ain't a bad position to be in. But we are not here to talk about the positives of stress—we are here to discuss its drawbacks.

And one of those drawbacks is what is known as stress-induced diabetes.

This is no Bigfoot, this stress-induced diabetes. In fact, numerous studies have found evidence of this, and it is worrisome. What happens when we become acutely stressed, is that the body triggers a hyperglycemic episode in order to get through the stressful episode (Sharma et al., 2022).

The issue is when this happens over long periods of time. Basically, chronic stress-related hyperglycemia leads to metabolic changes, which, along with other factors, can lead to insulin resistance. This is why chronically stressed out people are at a high risk of type-2 diabetes (Sharma et al., 2022).

Now we already know the risks associated with type-2 diabetes. But the fact that chronic stress can trigger it means that chronic stress is itself life-threatening.

Now let's tie everything together. When we do not get enough sleep, we become stressed. When we become stressed, our body responds by triggering a hyperglycemic state. Chronic stress can cause type-2 diabetes; chronic sleep deprivation can cause chronic stress; therefore, chronic sleep deprivation can cause type-2 diabetes.

So, yeah. Make sure you get enough sleep, folks. Because your blood sugar levels will be affected, and those effects can be deadly.

***

So much for the factors influencing our glucose levels. What we want to know now is, what sorts of benefits can we get from keeping those levels—well, *level*?

Just how healthy can we get by monitoring our blood sugar?

And the answer to that is—VERY.

Chapter 3:

The Long-Term Health Benefits of Maintaining Stable Glucose Levels

"Being healthy" means many things to many people. Some people might say that it means eating well and exercising but forget that mental health is just as important. Some people might even say the opposite: They might focus on mental health at the expense of their physical health, such as when people eat junk food to be happy.

But really, being healthy is something both physical and mental. It means being in the optimal condition that our bodies can possibly be in. Which sounds simple, but, alas, is insanely complicated.

There are just so many damn things that go into being healthy. And advice on how to achieve perfect health at this point is like a constant, static noise that shows no signs of abating.

With that in mind, we need to recognize that glucose regulation is not a one-size-fits-all cure-all for every disease known to man. It is not snake oil. Plenty of diets will claim to be just that, but since our bodies are so complicated, and health no less so, those diets will fall short of their claimed benefits and, more often than not, go the way of the dodo.

What we can claim about glucose regulation, however, is that there are certain health conditions which can be unlocked by virtue of our adopting this practice. And not just any, either— we are talking about, of course, preventing diabetes, but also gaining control of our weight, improving our focus, and preventing cardiovascular disease.

As I said in the previous chapter, taking control of our blood sugar is a very healthy choice. So that said, let's take a deep dive into some of these conditions, learn how they are related to blood sugar, and see if we can't figure out how to prevent them from happening.

Diabetes

We have already gone over type-2 diabetes in some detail earlier, but we are going to start off with a bit of a refresher.

This is, first off, the most common form of diabetes. You are at risk for it if you are overweight, or if you have a close relative who has it. If you do have it, you are at risk of heart disease, stroke, and both foot and eye problems, including blindness.

In short, this is not one of the illnesses you want. Having T2D, as it is called, means potentially a lifetime of managing your illness, which can include taking shots of insulin.

So how, then, do we make sure we do not wind up with T2D?

There are a few things. First off, if you lose even a modest amount of weight, you are helping yourself stave off T2D. As a matter of fact, by losing only between 5-7% of your bodyweight, you drastically reduce the possibility of getting the disease (National Institute of Diabetes and Digestive and Kidney Diseases (NIDDKD), 2019).

You should also get more exercise, as we have talked about. Even 30 minutes of exercise five days a week can be enough. And not only that, but you will feel better generally as a result (NIDDKD, 2019).

And, finally, there is the ever-reliable healthy eating that prevents this terrible disease from happening in the first place.

Which, okay, yes, I know none of this is new to us now. But we should take a second to think about what is being said here. Basically, we know that there is a connection between these three things and our blood sugar. We know that losing weight, exercising, and eating well helps balance our glucose levels. And we know that not doing so will put us at risk for T2D.

We also know what the risks are if we do develop T2D. Blindness and limb amputation are obviously at the far end of the spectrum, but neither of those come out of nowhere, either. Leading up to each of those is a lot of suffering.

What kind of suffering are we talking about? Dizziness. Lethargy. Visits to the doctor. Extreme thirst and frequent urination. Worrying about our symptoms.

All of that, plus, if coupled with not managing our symptoms, an increase in our total suffering, until, finally, we develop foot and eye problems.

Not exactly a walk in the park.

But for all that, T2D is a preventable disease, which means it is not necessary that we go through it. And all we have to do to keep it at arm's length is to make healthy choices most of the time. Not all the time, because that would be insane. But most of the time.

And if we can do that, then we are ensuring we do not have to go through the type of suffering that people with type-2 diabetes have to go through. Which means a whole myriad of problems, small and large, have been prevented because of the healthy choices we made.

And which, finally, means not just preventing diabetes, but ensuring a higher degree of flourishing in our day-to-day lives.

But we have talked about diabetes at length already. So, with that out of the way, we should move onto energy levels.

Fatigue

Fatigue in itself is not a bad thing. In fact, fatigue is perfectly natural—it just means being tired, after all.

So when we end a hard day of manual labor, work out, or even have a veggie day of doing nothing at all, we are probably going to feel tired. Chronic fatigue, however, is another beast entirely.

Now there are numerous causes of chronic fatigue. Many of them, however, can be linked back to poor habits (not counting the ones that arise from serious health problems). One of those causes, and the one most crucial for our purposes, is diabetes.

But just how linked to chronic fatigue is diabetes? Well, how about for a stat: A whopping 85% of people with chronic fatigue have diabetes. Which means that having the condition can affect how well we function in the day-to-day, performance-wise—considering how hard it is to function when chronically fatigued (Walker Family Care, n.d.).

"Okay, okay," I can hear you asking. "But what about those of us without diabetes? Does blood sugar impact our energy levels also?"

Well, as with many things food and diet-related, the evidence is inconclusive and largely in its infancy. But with the spirit of discovery in mind, we should go through what information we do have and see what we can't discover.

One interesting irony in all this is that the more "energy" we have in our blood, the less energetic we feel. In other words, hyperglycemia makes us feel tired. One study found that by increasing blood sugar in participants, memory and cognition were impaired, there was a decrease in how quickly they could process information, and they felt sadder and more anxious than they did prior to the hyperglycemic episode (The Levels Team, 2020).

Does this sound totally out to lunch? Well, consider how you tend to feel after you overeat. Say, Christmas. Do you feel super smart? Like you could run a marathon? Ready to work out and run around trying to keep up with toddlers?

No, you feel sluggish. Of course, you do. In fact, many of us might even have taken a bit of a nap after Christmas dinner. Or known someone who has.

Is it the case, then, do dips in blood sugar make us energetic?

Alas, no. Dips in blood sugar have basically the same effect. And by the way, this applies to dips in blood sugar at night too. One study found that nocturnal hypoglycemia meant that, after exercise the next day, participants were more likely to enter a state of fatigue and feel a general decrease in their well-being (The Levels Team, 2020).

And how about this for new information: A post-hyperglycemia dip, known as reactive hypoglycemia, is extra responsible for making you super tired. (The notorious "sugar crash," in other words.) But this generally happens as a result of eating foods that are high on the glycemic index. And, what's more, eating foods that are low GI can prevent episodes like this from happening, meaning that the solution is actually pretty simple (The Levels Team, 2020).

So, yeah, basically your blood sugar doing anything but staying at a reasonable and stable level is going to make you tired. Which means, if you have been keeping score, that people with absolutely no form of diabetes should consider how their blood glucose affects their energy levels, and which types of food (hint: low GI) they should consume in order to rectify this.

But let's get a bit more specific, just so there are no lingering questions.

First off, it is clear that merely choosing to eat different foods is not the simple proposition it sounds like. I am, of course, well aware that there is a profound psychological component to doing this. You have to change the way you think about food, how you interact with it, what you use it for. So, yes, changing your eating habits is a challenging proposition.

With regard to energy levels, then, many of us are locked into this much more metabolically destructive way of trying to get energy. For example, when we feel tired, we might go for an energy drink, or drink more coffee.

But this is not the way to have more consistent levels of energy most of the time. Diet, in fact, is the key ingredient when it comes to energy.

And how do we do that? Well for one, you might consider reducing your carb intake per meal. This will not work for everybody, as not everybody is sensitive to carbs in the same way. But if you know your body well enough and you know that carbs make you sleepy, then maybe consider lightening your carb load for a few meals and see what happens (The Levels Team, 2020).

You also might consider mixing up which carbs you do take in. So, maybe bread is what tuckers you out but pasta does not. Why not just go with pasta then? You can even try a banana, which, for some of us, is a great and profound source of energy.

Think, too, about some of the other things we have talked about with regard to glucose. Sleep, exercise, all these things affect our blood sugar levels. If we want to have energy, to stay awake throughout the day and not fight sleep, then we want to have a blood glucose level that is neither spiking nor dipping. We want to stay level to stay energized.

Which means what exactly?

Well, with regard to energy levels, people with diabetes need to worry about this especially. The connection between diabetes and fatigue is well-established and this means that, if you are diabetic, you have to be concerned with taking steps to protect yourself from fatigue.

But while we said earlier that the connection between blood glucose and energy is less clear for non-diabetics, there are still some signs that it might be worth thinking about. For example, given that dips and spikes both have caused fatigue in participant studies suggests that taking care to keep our blood glucose level could lead to our being more energetic throughout the day.

And there is still, as suggested earlier, some evidence from experience. The "sugar high" is well-known and particularly among those of us with young children in the family. We have all seen kids eat too much sugar, go crazy, and then have a nap afterwards.

So, all that together does hint at a chance that taking part in the glucose revolution will help keep us more active for longer periods. Which means better job performance, less stress, more time to be present for when we need to be.

And so, with that, it is time to move on.

Focus and Cognition

As we have moved along through this subject of blood glucose, we have found that our blood sugar impacts a host of systems, and everything else, in our bodies. But while we have touched on issues of cognitive decline and brain health, and how hyperglycemia in specific affects our ability to focus, we are going to take a deeper dive into this issue, to make sure no stone is left unturned.

Lest somebody accuse us of not being thorough.

Okay, starting from the top. We all lose our focus from time to time. We get into this or that situation, only to find that we do not have the ability to think as clearly as we did even just an hour before. Sometimes this is in an important situation, like one involving money; sometimes it is just a simple little annoyance, like when we are playing mini golf. (Although in fairness, mini golf can be wicked hard.)

There are obviously a billion reasons why this may be happening. But there is a chance this is connected to our blood glucose, as we will see.

Glucose, as it turns out, is our brain's primary fuel source. Evidence for this is by no means scant either: Participants in a study scored higher on cognitive skills when provided with a glucose load, as compared to the placebo. Memorization, in particular, seems to be affected by low glucose levels. And, what's more, as we perform complex mental tasks, like memorization, our blood glucose levels decrease from being used.

Basically, what happens is that when our blood sugar is too low, our brain cannot make the neurotransmitters, which is how our brain communicates with itself and our body. Basically, the neurons stop being able to send messages to one another. When we are in a state of hypoglycemia, there is a near-guarantee that we lose some of our cognitive function upon entering that state (Edwards, 2016).

Despite this, similarly to what we talked about earlier, too much glucose is not good for the brain either. One study apparently found that excess sugar led to our cells aging faster, while another found evidence of cognitive decline associated with high blood sugar (Edwards, 2016).

Nowhere is this clearer, by the way, than in people with diabetes. Long-term diabetics with high blood sugar levels can have such horrific things happen to them as their brain actually undergoing atrophy, for crying out loud. And not only that, but they can develop diseases which restrict blood flow to the brain, causing vascular dementia (Edwards, 2016).

One of the more interesting developments in this field involves an insulin nasal spray. How this works is not really important for our purposes, but what makes it interesting is that users performed better in a variety of cognitive tasks. So, while type-2 diabetes especially does horrific things to the brain, there is some hope of, not a total reversal, but some improvement (Edwards, 2016).

One of the ways in which they improved was in things like visual perceptions and spatial relationships, too (Edwards, 2016). Because, yes, how well you interact with your environment obviously begins with the brain.

But if that were true, then should we not see blood glucose having a more pronounced effect on athletes?

In fact, that does appear to be the case. But why is this?

Well, sports do require more mental focus than non-sports people often care to admit. And studies have shown that athletes who have ingested carbohydrates tend to perform better across all areas in the second halves of exercise-heavy games (Supersapiens, 2022). So, as far as contexts to look at this in, this one seems to be fruitful.

Soccer, for starters, has shown consistent results with regards to carbohydrate consumption and athletic performance. In fact, most studies have shown that carbs make soccer players play better in a variety of different areas.

In this case, since we are talking about soccer, we are talking about things like dribbling, shooting, and passing—the standard moves in the game. But on top of that, these effects seem to manifest where it counts the most: toward the end of a game, when players are exhausted enough to make silly mistakes.

Cycling is another area where the results are pretty well crystal clear. Hypoglycemia impairs neuromuscular performance, and so cyclists, who are in a near-constant state of movement, are especially affected by low blood sugar. Furthermore, performance during periods of up to three hours of moderately intense exercise seems to remain consistent when blood sugar is at a reasonable level.

And lastly, looking at tennis and other court sports—by the way, I have no idea if you, Dear Reader, are athletic in any way shape or form. But I never liked tennis. I guess I have always been sensitive to loud noises, and tennis matches tend to make such a racket.

Anyway.

Recall that earlier we were talking about how blood sugar helps us interact with our environment better? Well, the thing about court games, including fencing, by the way, is that they depend to an insanely high degree on accuracy. If you have ever seen a game of squash or racquetball, you will know exactly what I am talking about.

Well, court sports seemed to have been particularly affected by blood sugar. In fact, having ingested a sensible amount of carbs, even elite-level fencers and squash players were found to have more consistent peak power output, and were less likely to develop muscular tiredness (Supersapiens, 2022).

In summary, then: Since sports require us to have a uniquely good handle on our environments, and to focus on a single task with an uncommon degree of skill; and since blood sugar affects our brain's ability to think, send messages to itself and, therefore, make sense of our environment; blood sugar levels will have a disproportionately high influence on athletes.

It appears as though this is the case. In at least the three areas covered, blood sugar which was kept level and at a reasonable place was found to make these athletes perform better across multiple areas.

But what about those of us who are not athletes? Well, the reason I included them was because athletic competition is by its nature extreme. We are looking at cases of people who function well outside the norm, in an effort to see which of them is the most outside the norm.

So, yes, I understand all that. But since they require a high degree of functioning, and since their mental faculties have to be particularly attuned to the task they are performing, they are, I think, great examples to show how this or that influence tends to affect human beings in such and such an area.

I think, by looking at those sports, that we can see blood glucose does have a significant effect on the athletes performing them. And that if that is true for them, then sure it is true for you and me.

In other words, by the looks of things, controlling our blood glucose is, in addition to everything else, going to give us improved cognitive abilities. And, in having done so, increase our ability to succeed in a given environment; since that is, ultimately, what our brain is there to help us do.

But look, we all know this is not what we are here for. All this stuff about improved cognitive function is great, but we want to know the big one: *how does all of this affect weight loss?*

Weight Loss

Okay, a little bit of review here first: When our body digests food, it breaks it down into glucose. We need this for all sorts of bodily functions, from our brains to our muscles and everything in between.

Our pancreas is what produces insulin, which has to be present or else glucose will not be able to go into our cells. Not enough insulin means our blood sugar levels rise, and too much insulin means our blood sugar goes too low.

What we want to know is: What in this scenario or high, low, or level blood sugar, is the optimal set of conditions for weight loss?

One thing we might find is that hypoglycemia appears to result in weight loss. But this is mistaking cause for effect: hypoglycemia can happen when we eat too little. If we eat too little, we lose weight (Crider, 2023).

Hyperglycemia too appears to result in weight loss under some circumstances; although, under others, it appears to result in weight gain. In cases where it results in weight gain, this is because the extra energy in your body winds up being stored as fat. But if that extra energy does not wind up in the body's cells, then the body does not get the energy it needs and so winds up burning fat as a result (Crider, 2023).

In other words, it is a crapshoot. Your blood sugar goes wonky, your body weight either goes up or down. Your metabolism, in other words, appears to go out of whack with your blood sugar. And in order to make sure that we are losing weight, or at least increase our chances of doing so, we will want a stable, regular metabolism.

Keeping your blood sugar level means, in addition to all the other cool things we have been talking about, keeping your metabolism regular.

So, when we have an interest in losing weight, which, judging by the stats, most of us either do or should, then we need to—surprise, surprise—think about what we are eating. We need to make sure that we are not eating foods that cause our blood glucose to spike or dip so that we can have a stable metabolism, in addition to calorie restricting and exercising. Those things together are what result in weight loss.

And by the way, as far as calorie restricting: notice that there are consequences to hypoglycemic episodes. Cognitive impairments being one of them. So calorie restriction is a delicate procedure because we need to also make sure that our bodies are not becoming less functioning as a result.

But, yes, in addition to everything, focusing on keeping our blood glucose level is an essential part to any weight loss strategy.

***

So, there you have it. The body is dependent on glucose for a wide variety of things, which means that keeping that blood sugar level will lead to improvements across all kinds of different areas of our lives.

But despite that, we still do not know how to pull this off. For example, what might a glucose meal plan look like? How does one even begin to know how to monitor one's glucose levels?

How the heck does a person even start to exercise or plan stress-reduction strategies to keep those glucose levels stable?

Well, hurry on, Dear Reader. Because that is exactly where we are off to next.

Chapter 4:

Practical Strategies for Glucose

Management

Now, it is time to get into the nitty-gritty.

Because at this point it should be clear that we have a solid theoretical base on which to make a plan. We know what blood sugar is, why we need it, all the basics. (Or, well, enough of the basics. Let's not get ahead of ourselves here).

So, with that in mind, we are going to jump into the practical side. We are going to go over how to monitor our glucose levels, what kind of exercise we can do to keep them stable, what kind of meal plans we might adopt—the whole gamut.

This is what we trained for, ladies and gentlemen. Onward and upward.

Continuous Glucose Monitors

We have talked an awful lot about how important it is to keep our blood glucose at a reasonable level. But, as you may have noticed, barring some sort of extra sensory perception, there does not seem to be any way to intuit what our blood glucose levels are.

Of course, when they get seriously out of whack, then we for sure notice. The dizziness or the confusion, the fatigue or whatever symptom we have—we notice then, for sure.

But without our levels going awry to that degree, how do we know where our glucose levels are at? Is there some sort of a machine that can give us the numbers? Some sort of... Continuous glucose monitoring device?

Okay, I have played my hand, and yes, there is such a device. In fact, continuous glucose monitoring means doing just that: using a device to give you real-time numbers on where your glucose levels are sitting. With it, you can check the (estimated) blood sugar levels at any time, and use that information to help plan your workouts, eating habits, the works (NIDDKD, 2023).

So, what is it? And how does it work?

The CGM, as it is known, has three parts. First, there is a part that is inserted under your skin. (I know, ouch—but how else are you supposed to know literally anything about your blood?) This part goes on your stomach or your arm, and has a sticky part that helps it stay there. But if this is not to your liking, there is also a version which is planted inside your body. Either way, what happens is these sensors read the amount of glucose in your cells, which should roughly correlate to how much glucose is in your blood.

After that, there is a transmitter. This part wirelessly sends information about your glucose to the third part, which is a software program you can keep on your smartphone. That way, you get information from your cells, through the transmitter right to your phone, for you to read at your leisure.

Now with that said, there are different versions of these devices, which store and transmit information differently. So, the "real-time" devices are the ones which send information to your phone. But there are also "intermittent-scan" versions which do a continuous monitor, but which need to be scanned by your smartphone so you can read the information. And finally, there is also a version which sends updates to your doctor, but this type is typically only worn for a limited time (NIDDKD, 2023).

No matter which type you wear, however, you will be wearing it all the time. This means it does not come off when you are sleeping or exercising, nor when you are showering. This way it can track all kinds of things, such as the types of food and beverages you are consuming, what your workouts are doing to your glucose levels, and what happens to your glucose during sleep.

You can also get an app which sounds an alarm when your blood glucose gets to dangerous levels, either too high or too low. If this alarm goes off, it is important that you get help right away, because your blood glucose has officially reached a level of concern.

As for benefits, these are probably clear, but we will go over them anyway. Obviously, you can monitor your blood glucose consistently, which will help give you the information you need to make healthy choices. This means, hopefully, having fewer emergencies.

But also, for people with diabetes who have to get their fingers pricked all the time at the doctor's office, that is no longer necessary (NIDDKD, 2023). Which is great, because getting your finger pricked sucks big time.

Which does not, however, mean that the finger pricks have become totally obsolete. There are a few issues with the monitors, which we will discuss here.

One thing is pretty obvious, given that we are talking about technology here— it has a tendency to fail. This machine is no different. There will be times when the machine is in error, and for a variety of different reasons. When this happens, a fingerpick will be necessary to compare with what the machine is suggesting, to see if maybe a replacement is in order. A fingerpick can additionally be necessary if you have changed your insulin dose or if your GM alarm has gone off (NIDDKD, 2023).

Returning to the issue of technology failing over time, these machines will need to be replaced either whole or in part, at some point after first using them. There are disposable sensors, too, which need to be replaced every week or so, although some of the implantable ones can last up to six months. The transmitters too can act up, same as the app on your smartphone. Either way, one of the three parts of your CGM can fail at any time and will therefore need to be fixed or replaced in order for you to continue continuously monitoring your glucose.

Another thing too: Sometimes people's skin reacts poorly to the machine. You can get itchy or see redness, or any other symptoms typically associated with allergy. And, finally these machines tend to cost more than a standard glucose meter, which is something to think about (NIDDKD, 2023).

And what about this other fancy thing—the artificial pancreas?

Well, this is basically an insulin delivery system that is inserted into the body, coupled with CGM. The CGM notes when your blood sugar has spiked, the insulin delivery system delivers insulin, and thus you have an artificial system doing the work of one standard pancreas (NIDDKD, 2023).

Now, all of this is fine and dandy, you might be saying. But so far this has all been about a system which assists people with diabetes in monitoring their blood glucose, which for them is a much more dire situation than for people who aren't affected by it. Is there any reason to believe that such a system would benefit those of us without diabetes?

The reality is that there are several companies which appear to believe there is such a benefit and are marketing their CGMs as a result. Which is likely why you may have heard of continuous glucose monitoring in the first place.

The question is whether or not the research supports this. And, as usual with this sort of thing, the results are not exactly in.

Let's start with the good news: One published study found that people without diabetes did not tend to have blood sugar problems (Shmerling, 2021). Now, if we really think about that, that's like saying that people without cancer do not tend to have life-threatening tumors. So, it is a bit of a tautology.

But on the other hand, it does call into question the usefulness of something like this for people without blood sugar problems. And, given how expensive these products can be, that might be a significant hurdle in our ability to recommend them in good conscience.

This is especially so since, as of 2021, there exist no studies which show that continuous glucose monitoring leads to better health outcomes for people without diabetes (Shmerling, 2021). Which, of course, does not mean that they do not promote good health amongst that cohort, but that there is no reason to think so, if we lean toward peer-reviewed science as the golden standard by which to measure truthfulness.

That being said, there are several reasons why someone might be interested in obtaining these results, despite the current dearth of evidence.

To begin with, it might be a useful way to tell if you are developing diabetes. Even prediabetics tend to have high blood sugar, just not enough for them to be considered diabetic. Testing your glucose would be a good way of detecting even prediabetes then. And, in fact, it is recommended that healthy people get their blood sugar tested every three years anyway, to make sure they are not developing either of these conditions (Shmerling, 2021).

But also consider that we have talked at length about all the ways in which our blood sugar affects us even without being diabetic. We have talked so far about mood stabilization, maximizing performance, and a whole host of other things. It might be that using one of these machines helps us to get a better understanding of where we are health-wise, so we can take steps to plan our meals and workouts and everything else, all in the service of reaching our potential.

And yet, we still haven't answered the question: Should a non-diabetic, who is interested in glucose control as a wellness practice, use a CGM?

Unfortunately, the answer is going to disappoint you. Because there really is no way of knowing, right now, whether or not a non-diabetic can benefit from one of these machines.

This is for a variety of reasons. One, obviously, is that there is not enough evidence to say that this will benefit non-diabetics. But additionally, it is not clear that these machines can offer information that we would not get from using the glycemic index to plan our meals, just as an example. What exactly would we gain from getting real-time updates on our blood sugar, particularly when non-diabetics tend to have healthy, stable blood glucose in the first place?

Remember, the whole point of this book is to discuss healthy eating and exercise habits related to glucose and carb intake, which can help us become healthier, better focused, and much more. Our focus really is on food and exercise, not pretending as though glucose monitoring requires the kind of constant attention that people with diabetes need to practice in order, frankly, to stay alive.

That being said, every one of us is a different beast. For some people, being able to monitor their blood glucose on their phone might be a way of asserting control over their health. If you can see the number, then it is not hidden; if it is not hidden, then it is not totally out of your control.

And, of course, there are a whole host of other reasons why someone might benefit from gaining access to that information. Which means, as usual, that the best course of action is to talk to your doctor. Tell them what your concerns are, what your goals are, and why you think you would benefit from using one of these machines.

Your doctor will know best whether or not this is a good idea. And if you take that information in with humility and grace, then you might have a better idea yourself whether you really need to use one of these machines.

Just remember your goals, keep your health in mind, and everything will turn out just fine.

So much for continuous glucose monitors. Next up, we need to focus on body movement; in specific, the kinds of exercises we need to do to keep that blood glucose in a healthy range, maximize our potential, and reap the rewards of good health.

Exercise

Alright, first things first: if you are an American reading this book, there is a good-to-fair chance that you are not getting nearly enough exercise.

How good is that chance, exactly? Well, according to the CDC, only 28% of Americans are meeting that threshold (Porterfield, 2023).

Meeting that threshold means, as an average person, that you are getting 150 minutes per week of aerobic exercise at a moderate intensity; and doing weight training at least twice a week. Of Americans surveyed, most of the exercise was being done in the West, while the South was doing the least (Porterfield, 2023).

These are not great numbers, alas. Exercise is so important that not doing it is really just sentencing yourself to a lifetime of ill-health. The benefits, then, are extraordinary, meaning everything from improved mood to improved cognitive function, to fewer physical health issues overall.

So, when I write this section saying that you, the Reader, should exercise, I know that it is likely you are groaning over the possibility. And I do not blame you one bit! What is better, in the short-term, pleasure-wise, than popping on a baseball game, opening a bag of chips, and drinking a few beers with some friends?

What I am saying is, I totally get it. Exercise is work, and human beings like to avoid work. It is in our nature.

But this is a book about health, dammit. And exercise is healthy—dammit. So, we are going to talk about its benefits, we are going to talk about what it does for your blood sugar, and we are going to talk about which exercises you should be doing to achieve the results you want.

Whether you take this advice is up to you. But I hope that by the end of this section, you will have been persuaded that this is worth doing.

And by the way, if you already exercise? That is fantastic. Consider this affirmation that you are doing the right thing. And see if maybe some of these workouts might help you along too.

By way of preliminaries then, what does exercise entail?

Exercise entails doing strenuous activity for a period of time, with the intention of improving your fitness. That is all. Within the domain of exercise, there are a bunch of different activities, and different classes of activity, which you can do to achieve fitness.

Now, if you are someone who does not exercise, the question of where to begin can seem daunting. Especially when you go into a gym, there are so many things to choose from, many of which seem vaguely dangerous.

Regardless of familiarity with the machines, the weights, and everything else, if you do not exercise or have not in a while, then you really should start light. You do not even have to use a gym to do this—you can go for a slow walk, for example, or even dust and vacuum your apartment. Not exactly a workout, but it will get the blood moving and introduce you to the idea of moving your body around (Diabetes Care, 2018).

If this is too little for you, or if you feel comfortable moving onto moderate exercise, then by all means, do so! You can go for a bike ride, a jog, swim or even dance. And if you feel up to something more vigorous, you could go running or play tennis.

Notice so far, we have not even mentioned the idea of going to a gym. That is because the gym is not essential for exercising; it is just a really convenient way to do so.

Remember over COVID when nobody could go to the gym? People would fill up buckets with water, place a broom handle through the bucket handles, and then use that instead of a barbell. There are all kinds of ways you can exercise without even leaving your house. So, if the gym is not for you, do not worry; there are plenty of other things you can do.

That said, the gym really is a convenient way to work out. Once you get the hang of the machines and get over the idea of people seeing you exercise, there are so many ways to get you fit in that one location.

Stationary bikes and treadmills are great for your cardio. You can program them to adjust their difficulty over time, which helps make the workout more interesting. These are great, solitary exercises too, so you can put on music (on headphones—do not be the guy who blasts his music for everyone else to hear), zone out and go for a run for as long as you like.

The weight machines might be a tad intimidating, but they tend to have diagrams on them, so you know how they work. These diagrams will tell you which muscles are being worked out also, which you should use as a guide to make sure you are using the machine properly. If it says it is working out your chest and you feel it somewhere else, you may want to adjust your posture, for example, to get the most out of the machine.

Posture is a key component of strength training, by the way. You will want to make sure your back is straight, with your shoulders pulled back and your chest out slightly. Anything else will probably hurt your back, and if you get hurt working out, you could be in a lot of trouble.

It is always important to stay safe when exercising. After all, you want to continue to do this week after week, ideally for the rest of your life. Hurting yourself will interfere with that.

With regard to the free weights: They are in some ways preferable to the machines. They actually wind up working out more of your body than just the muscle you are focusing on, largely because your posture is a more significant factor during these workouts. And any workout which uses more than one muscle group is going to be your friend, especially if you are doing full-body workouts.

Which, by the way, is probably what you will be doing at first, maybe two or three days a week. If you do more than that, you will probably split up your muscle groups; so, for example, you will work out your upper body one day, then your lower body the next, giving your upper body a rest.

As far as how a workout itself is structured (and yes, there is a structure), it essentially goes like this: You begin by doing some warmup exercises; then you do your workout; then you do some cool down exercises. Just like a story, with a beginning, a middle, and an end.

Warm-up exercises are important, because you are about to put your body through stress, and you want to make sure you do not hurt yourself. But there is more to it than that! Warm-up exercises also increase your flexibility and range of motion, improve your performance, and increase blood flow and oxygen (Cronkleton, 2019).

Of warm-up exercises, there are two basic ones that we will cover here. The first is called the dynamic warm-up, which basically gets you ready for a high-intensity workout. This involves things like squats and pushups, and in their own way improves your strength and coordination (Cronkleton, 2019).

Static stretching is the other one. For these, you stretch a muscle and then hold it for a time. This gets your muscles ready for a workout and helps prevent injury (Cronkleton, 2019).

The workout itself will be whatever you have decided to do that day. It might be arms, back, legs, full-body, whatever. It might be machines, free weights, or even bodyweight. But this is where you get most of your work done.

Some people like to work out by themselves, others with a partner. Some exercises, especially bench press, are best done with a partner, to help prevent injury. Myself, I like to work out alone, which means I may have to substitute bench press for a chest workout involving a dumbbell in each hand. These substitutions are totally fine, so long as they work out the same muscle group.

For cooldowns, I like to do a bit of yoga afterward. Just some light stuff, stretching a bit, relaxing, letting my heart rate come down. After about fifteen minutes of that, I consider the workout over and usually have a veggie protein shake.

Now, we already talked earlier about the benefits exercising has on your blood sugar levels. The main takeaway, for me, was that in the long-term, exercise helps keep your blood sugar stable, even though it leads to short-term spikes.

The key takeaway from this section then, should be which exercises can be done in order to pull this feat off. We should structure our workouts in such a way that we make sure not to hurt ourselves, and we get the results we are looking for, which is especially possible when combined with healthy dietary choices.

Now, for those of us who struggle with keeping up a workout schedule, there is some good news ahead: There are plenty of apps which are designed for this exact purpose.

The number of apps which do this is too many to list all of them here, and a full-scale review of even a bunch falls outside the scope of this book. But I will say that I have used apps like Nike Training Club with a high degree of success but have also been using an app called Workout which is almost miraculous in its ability to provide a weekly structure of individualized workouts.

So, yes, getting into the specifics here: Many of these apps will give you a schedule, designed around how many days you want to exercise, how comfortable you are in a gym or at home, whether or not you use weights—the whole shebang. They will give you a list of exercises to do on these days, which, on many apps, can be subbed out for other ones.

If apps are your thing, then I wholeheartedly recommend them. They have been fantastic at getting my own workouts on a solid schedule, which is good for me since I tend to slip away over time. (Which also totally happens—you get in, you like the exercise, you slip a little, you slip a lot, you get out... Just so long as you pick up and start again, do not sweat it. We all do it!)

All in all, then, there are plenty of places, methods, and everything else that you can use to help get your body moving. Whichever one works for you, app or no app, at home or the gym, weights or bodyweight—if it works, then it works.

Getting into the habit of exercising will be one of the best choices you ever made, if you have not already. And it is an indispensable tool for managing your blood glucose levels.

But exercising will not amount to a hill of beans without proper nutrition. So, with that in mind, it is time to start talking about what we should eat.

Diet in Practice

And speaking of what we should eat...

I have always been a big movie person. Especially horror movies. Every new one that comes out, I am the first one in line. I cannot get enough of them—ghosts, slashers, you name it. If it is a scary movie, I am 100% there.

But my favorite of all of them is the zombie movie. I have seen them all: *Night Of The Living Dead, Day Of The Dead, Zombie Flesheaters*... Ones that come from America, from Italy, even some Spanish and Australian ones. I have seen every season of *The Walking Dead* and *Fear The Walking Dead*. I am, in a word, obsessed.

So, you can imagine that after all these years of watching zombie movies, I have pretty well seen them all. And while there is a certain pride in that, I can also attest to the fact that the scenarios in these movies have become terribly dull.

For example, the first time I watched an Italian zombie movie, I was enthralled by how crazy and bizarre the whole thing was. It seemed like a whole new world! The ridiculous acting, the jungle settings, the number of laws broken in the making of those pictures... It was a veritable lifestyle choice for me, and for years, I was hooked.

But after about thirty or so of those, even one I am seeing for the first time feels dull, predictable. Even the craziest concepts get an eye roll. *Zombies Vs Rednecks, Redneck Zombies, Zombies From The Planet Xenon*, none of them attract my attention. And so, I have been desperately looking for a zombie movie with a fresh concept, wondering if maybe my time with the zombie movie has come to a close.

Then, of course, a friend of mine said there was a new type of zombie movie I had never heard of.

"You know how zombie movies are all parodies of things?" he said. "Like how *Dawn Of The Dead* is about consumerism and *Land Of The Dead* is about President Bush?"

"Yeah...?"

"Well, this one is about diet culture. See, zombies normally eat people, right? But people pollute their bodies with all kinds of drugs and processed foods and stuff. So, the zombies would presumably get real sick from eating us."

"Aren't zombies already dead though?"

"Shush, it doesn't matter. Anyway, what happens in this one is that zombies shun unhealthy food, i.e., people. And they start a sort of commune, where they share workloads and spread the wealth around..."

"But what do they eat?"

"What's that?"

I said, "What do they eat?"

"Oh," my friend said. "In this one they're vegetarians."

I couldn't believe this. "Vegetarian zombies? So what, they eat carrots and salad?"

"No, they wander into farmer's fields and eat the crops."

"Corn?"

"No, not corn."

"Then what?" I said, exasperated.

"*Grrraaaaiiiinssssss...*"

I know, I know. Great joke. You can thank me later.

Anyway, back to the task at hand.

So, in this section we are going to swing on back to the low GI diet, doing a bit of a refresher plus putting together a meal plan. Since we decided that the monitoring systems were of ambiguous utility, it is important that we pay attention to what types of foods we are ingesting as a way to control our blood sugar.

Couple it with exercise, and we will be some lean, mean machines.

First things first: Since we are in the market for a balanced, nutritional way of losing weight and staying or getting healthy, the low GI diet is a good one to use. It means eating lots of whole grains, fruits, vegetables, and lean proteins like fish and chicken. Because it allows for a slower release of glucose, you are less likely to feel hungry soon after eating a meal, which prevents overeating (Chalicha, 2022).

Now, we know that eating low GI foods is good for your blood sugar. But because of this, it is also good for your heart health, since there is a strong connection between blood sugar problems and heart disease. Because low GI foods tend to be high in fiber, and low in saturated fats, they help to both lower blood sugar levels and reduce inflammation, both of which help to keep our hearts healthy (Chalicha, 2022).

How do we know if a certain food is high- or low-GI? The list is of course available online, and I have already provided a version of that in this book. But there are factors which influenced a food's GI, some of which include: the level of processing; the ripeness of fruit, in that ripened fruit has a higher GI score; preparation, such as whether we deep fry something; how much, and what kind of, dressing we put on it; and the type of starch in the food (Chalicha, 2022).

All of which should do as a refresher for the low-GI diet, but in case you feel like you are forgetting something, well, this is a book; you can always go back to the section on the GI diet and read it again.

Still, suffice it to say, the GI diet appears to be a healthy one, and we know roughly how t0 determine which foods are included in this particular diet, which is great. But now we should get onto the actual meal plan (Chalicha, 2022).

DAY ONE

Okay, for this day we are going to start off breakfast with some scrambled eggs, smoked salmon, and whole wheat bread. This way we are getting in our protein and our carbs are coming from whole wheat, not white bread.

For lunch, we will have some spicy beef noodle lettuce wraps.

The lettuce wrap, in case you have not heard of it, is a fantastic substitute for your usual wrap. Lettuce has basically no calories, which means you do not really have to calculate it on top of everything you put in it. And, surprisingly enough, it works really well as a wrap. You can even use it as a substitute for buns!

For a snack, we should get in some low-fat fruit yogurt. Lots of people have different preferences for yogurt, that is perfectly fine. If you prefer to use plain yogurt and throw some fruit in yourself, that is fine too. Personally, I go blueberry.

Finally, our dinner is going to be baked chicken with couscous.

Already we should notice that even going on a low-GI diet, we do not have to sacrifice flavor or enjoyment. This is all good food, it tastes great, and there is plenty of variety.

DAY TWO

Breakfast, today, we are going to start off with oats and honey. Instant oats, if you remember, are not low-GI. But luckily, steel cut oats are cheap and super healthy. And what is better than oats with honey?

For lunch: lentil soup with a slice of wholemeal bread. Now, for soups we have a bit of a tricky situation. Some of us like to make soup, some of us like to buy soup. Making soup is a great way to take control of how healthy your soup is, but, alas, it can be time consuming. Just remember, if you buy your soup from the store, that you should check the labels first. You will want to make sure that what you are buying is not, say, packed to the gills with salt.

For a snack today, we are going to have mixed nuts and seeds, and a medium-sized pear. Those of you with nut allergies should have a good idea of what to substitute nuts with, but in case you do not, it is recommended that you look into ways of replacing them. Maybe leaning on seeds more? It is up to you.

Finally for dinner, a seafood stir fry with brown rice. Stir fries are insanely easy to make, and brown rice can be made quite quickly. Honestly, this might be my favorite meal in this whole plan.

DAY THREE

Alright, for breakfast, we are going to go with the repeat here and have scrambled eggs, smoked salmon, and wholegrain toast.

But check this out: For lunch, we are going to do what are called Vietnamese lettuce wraps.

So, we have already talked about the benefits of the lettuce wrap over a traditional wrap. But the idea of putting Vietnamese food into any style of wrap was new to me, at least until recently. And let me tell you, it is fantastic.

First off, Vietnamese food is amazing. There are so many great things to try if you have not already. The most famous is probably the Bahn Mi sandwich, but there are a bunch of different soups and salads and everything else, and all of them are great.

Basically, all we are going to do here is pick out whichever Vietnamese food we like and which would work well in a wrap, and then wrap it up in lettuce. It sounds simple (because, yeah, it is) but seriously: so worth it.

For a snack today, we are going to have low-fat yogurt. Yogurt is great without anything in it, so today we are going to try it without throwing anything extra in. But of course, if you would prefer to chuck some fruit in there, then do it by all means.

For dinner today, we are going to go with the ultimate post-workout meal. We are going to have roast chicken with sweet potatoes and broccoli.

This is the kind of thing athletes eat for a reason. Lots of protein, and it fills you up. And if it sounds plain, well, you already had a Vietnamese lettuce wrap. You can't have exciting food for every meal of the day.

DAY FOUR

Breakfast here is a return to oats, but this time we are going to toss in some blueberries and a bit of low fat milk, or milk substitute. Blueberries really are one of the great foods of the world, by the way. They are so good for you, and can be put in everything from oats to, oddly enough, salad. In fact, a salad with lettuce, spinach, blueberries, and cheese is a great meal.

But I digress.

Lunch is going to be an interesting one. Lots of us know chicken and rice soup, but what about a rice soup without the chicken?

This is probably one we will have to make ourselves. Fortunately, making soup is fun. And you can make a boatload of it to last you a super long time, and for very little money.

The only thing to remember is that rice can be tricky! White rice, jasmine, none of those things are low-GI. We want brown rice to make this diet plan work, which, fortunately, can be found everywhere rice is sold.

For a snack today, we are going to have my personal favorite, the fruit smoothie. Peach and mango is a recommendation from me, but obviously you can mix and match, either with fresh or frozen fruits. Add some low-fat yogurt for consistency, and if you really want to, you can throw in some honey.

What I do is, I get two big bags of frozen fruits from the grocery store; one of them is usually some kind of mix, like an Arctic mix or a summertime mix, and the other is something like raspberries or strawberry rhubarb. But the trick is that every week I get two different kinds of frozen fruit, so I have some variety.

I tend to mix mine with bananas, but you do whatever you want. I also use water and no milk. Again, your call.

For dinner, we will go with a grilled swordfish and a quinoa salad. Swordfish is probably the best fish, if you ask me. (It is even good on sandwiches.) So, dinner tonight is going to be amazing.

DAY FIVE

Now that we have a bit of a handle on the kinds of foods we are talking about and why we should be eating them, we can pretty well breeze through the next few days, since most of the foods will be repeats.

Breakfast today is oats, blueberries and honey; lunch will be low-fat chicken noodle soup; snack is a fruit smoothie; dinner is grilled salmon with broccoli and chickpeas.

DAY SIX

Breakfast will be oats with blueberries, skimmed milk and walnuts; lunch is brown rice salad with tuna or chicken; for a snack, we will do another fruit smoothie; and for dinner, a steak stir fry over brown rice.

DAY SEVEN

Alright folks, this is it: the main event!

Breakfast will be porridge with honey; lunch is quinoa salad with greens and beans; snack is a fruit smoothie with nuts or seeds;

and dinner is chicken with olives, sun dried tomatoes, and wholemeal pasta.

***

So, all in all, what have we learned here?

Well, hopefully we have a decent idea of what a low-GI diet looks like, because if we plan on continuing with it, then we will likely want to improvise our own versions in the future; unless, that is, you want to use this seven-day schedule for literally the rest of your life.

With this then, you can mix and match, figure out what your favorites are, sub out the things you do not like, but in the end, you will be eating the kinds of things that keep your blood sugar steady, and stop the endless spike-and-dip cycle which so many of us are on.

But altogether, I hope that by now we have a good idea of how we can and should handle our lifestyle choices, so that we can take better control of our blood glucose. Obviously, there is much more we could have discussed, so consider this a sensible primer. And if it interests you, then I fully encourage you to continue your investigations.

Which brings us to our next chapter—because while we have talked about the kind of broad-stroke, one-size-fits-all nutrition and exercise plans, this is, alas, not going to work for everybody. Different people have different dietary needs, which means most of us will have to personalize our meal plans, our exercise routines—the works.

Turn the page then, and let's figure out how to pull that off together.

Chapter 5:

Customizing Glucose

Management Strategies

No two people are exactly the same.

I know, I know. Quite the thought, right? But while this seems like a truism, it is nonetheless true that we see one-size-fits-all solutions everywhere. People are constantly being told that whatever problems you face, there is one simple thing that needs to be added into your life, the economy, the political sphere, whatever—and everything will turn out for the best.

Unfortunately, things are more complicated than that.

All around us is evidence of diversity. Look at any other animal, if it makes you feel better, and look at the varieties there are in that species. It could be something like an insect, maybe a housefly. There are some that are bigger, some that are smaller; some that are faster, some that are slower. Infinite variety within one single type of organism.

Why would it be any different for us humans? We are all of the same species, but within that species is an infinite variety. Hair color, eye color, ability, intelligence—all of it, put together in a single person, to create something utterly unique.

Alright, I am getting a little poetic here. But the point is that we have been talking a lot about what to eat, and how much of it to eat, yet we have not addressed the simple fact that every person is not only unique, but as a result, also has a unique set of needs. This is true not just of our wants and desires, but our dietary needs as well.

What do we do about that?

It turns out, we can just create our own meal plans.

In this chapter, we are going to go over what it means to create a personalized meal plan. Not just how to do it, but why, and what kind of hurdles we might encounter along the way. We are also going to talk about whether we should use dietitians, or do it totally on our own.

And we are going to do this because getting away from the kind of universal prescriptions for health is important. So, suit up, dig in, and let's get ready to learn about customized meal plans—starting with everything we need to know about dietitians.

Dietitians: What We Need to Know

First off: What the heck is a dietitian, anyway?

A dietitian is a medical professional who specializes in food nutrition. "Nutritionist" is another word that gets thrown around a lot, and there is some confusion about which is which, depending on where you live. In some areas, both words are used; in some areas, they mean different things.

For simplicity's sake, I am going to use "dietitian" to mean the kind of medical professional I have described above.

So why are we talking about them?

Well, for a lot of people, these experts are the perfect gateway to realizing their nutrition goals. They work with health professionals across the spectrum, from nurses and doctors, to social workers, and even speech language pathologists. They also have advocacy roles in terms of how they influence law and policy around nutrition, promotion of this or that consumer product, and on (College of Dietitians of Alberta n.d.).

As far as what this means for you as an individual, seeing one is essentially a consultation where they give you practical advice on how to meet your health needs. But since we are here for some specifics, here are some of the ways a dietitian can help you:

Maybe you are struggling with some type of illness, like say blood pressure problems, or Crohn's disease. A dietitian can help coach you through all the necessary changes in your diet and lifestyle, so you can implement them and achieve the health outcome you have been looking for (College of Dietitians of Alberta, n.d.).

Maybe you are the kind of person who is confused by how to read nutrition labels; or maybe you have just been given terrible advice on what those fancy words mean. (For example: the adage not to eat anything you have trouble pronouncing is ridiculous.) A dietitian can help you understand the complicated world of food labels, how to shop for groceries in a smarter way, and even how to save money doing so.

Maybe you and/or your family is/are looking to lose some weight and become healthier. Well, a dietitian excels in this! They can, and this is crucial for us, help to develop an individualized plan which will help you reach those goals.

But how exactly does the process work?

Well, the first thing a dietitian might do is assess your eating routine. In doing so, they can get a handle on what you are not doing, and therefore what you should be doing, to improve your health outcomes (Sass, 2015).

Before they give the kind of concrete advice that will help you reach your goals, they may try and figure out which kind of plan would work best for you. They may try and figure out, for example, if you are the kind of person who responds well to a heavily structured plan, with personalized meal plans and grocery lists and the like; or, if maybe you are the kind of person who works best with concrete goals, and feels more comfortable improvising toward them. Either way, if you are seeing a dietitian, you will want to be up-front about which of these styles works best for you. Remember, you are there with goals in mind, and not being open and honest will not help you get there (Sass, 2015).

Some dietitians will encourage follow-ups that may include weekly check-ins for a month, just as an example. If that does not work, the dietitian may ask you to keep a food journal, perhaps as frequently as every day. Either way, the dietitian will want information that shows whether the plan is working and what needs to be tweaked. If you eat out often, for example, then a diet that requires you to cook at home is not going to work for you, and the dietitian will want this information to assess your progress.

Additionally, the plan they have come up with might be making you feel sluggish or sick. This happens—the human body is kind of a stupid organism sometimes, at least from the perspective of medical science. Often, something that should work produces the opposite result, and the plan has to be changed. Dietitians are sensitive to this kind of thing and should have no problem adjusting the plan to make sure you do not feel like crap (Sass, 2015).

One thing that has improved as a result of the COVID-19 pandemic is that medical professionals do a lot of meetings either over the phone or through Skype or Zoom. Dietitians are no different: Instead of having to go into an office, wait a gazillion hours around a bunch of people coughing and sneezing and complaining to the secretary, only to find out the doctor is running late and will not be able to see you for an hour, you can just hop online or on the phone and do everything basically on time, and within a reasonable timeframe (Sass, 2015). So, there is that too, which makes signing up for one much easier.

Another thing too is that some dietitians will actually meet you at your home. That way they can look through your fridge, take an assessment of what you like to keep around and what you should throw out, as well, perhaps, even cook with you, to show you how this or that thing is done.

Now obviously some of us would not enjoy that. (I am one of those people.) So, if that is not going to work for you, just make sure you let the dietitian know where and what your boundaries are. They are willing and able to work around your needs and desires and level of comfortability.

Either way, the point here is that the dietitian is someone whose job it is to help you get on the right track, to meet your goals health-wise. As you can see from everything above, they are willing to adapt to your schedule, needs, whatever, in order to help you get there.

As far as coming up with a personalized meal plan, this is probably the best way to do it. You are finding someone with the right credentials, who knows how to make this work for you, and will tailor their recommendations to your preferences.

Are there downsides? In a word: yes.

The fact of the matter is that not every insurance plan covers dietitians. Which means that, if you are American and reading this, the dietitian might be an expensive option, and you might not be able to afford that.

And before you get jealous over Canadians, I cannot find anything which says that any provincial health plan covers dietitians. So, this might be an expensive option for the Canadians in the crowd also.

There is also the chance that going through a professional who will tell you what and how to eat is a little, well, *patronizing*. Some of us might feel our backs get up, like, we are saying, "I don't need anybody to tell me how to eat. I can just figure that out for myself."

And that is fair! But before we proceed with that line of thinking, I would like to tell you a story.

I grew up in a small town. The culture there was very much of the, "You leave me alone, I leave you alone" variety. Which was nice, but there was also this strongly-held animosity with big cities that was occasionally to their disadvantage.

I think what it was, was that people were tired of being looked down upon. Which is a real phenomenon, where city people think small towns are filled with utter morons who cannot even read. But how some people in this small town responded to this, was by acting as though they had superior skills or knowledge just by virtue of being themselves.

I will give you an example. One of my neighbors was an old man who had spent all his life on a farm. When someone close to him used a word he did not understand, he would go on a rant about how school was useless. Everything he knew was more important than what could be taught behind the brick walls of the education system.

He was doing this because he did not like having a hole poked in his ego, I am sure. Instead of admitting that some people might know more than him, or that the choices he made or had to make were not always in his best interest, or even doing something to better himself, he just attacked the thing, person, whatever it was that was superior to him.

The worst case of all this though was a woman named Cheryl. She lived around the corner, was about thirty-six years old, and had a horrible attitude. If the old farmer did not respond well to having his ego penetrated, she was only that much worse. The slightest hint that she was not the queen of all existence, and she would fly off the handle, usually with a flurry of insults.

Her husband, meanwhile, was a nice man named Harold. And it was through him that everyone learned Cheryl had developed a weird growth on her head.

"I told her," he said, "to get that thing looked at. Sort of on her forehead, you understand? Right by her hairline? It doesn't look like much, but she should at least get a second opinion."

Of course, Cheryl was sure she knew everything anyone needed to know. So, she refused to heed his advice, saying she knew what it was, that it was just a new mole. Doctors, she said, just made everything more complicated than it needed to be. And after all those years spent indoors reading, what the hell did they know anyway?

A few weeks went by and it was clear to everyone that this was not just some mole. In fact, one of the doctors who lived in town, Dr. Roberts, saw her come into the convenience store and told her as much, to which she responded by grabbing a handful of chocolate bars and throwing them at him.

When Harold heard about this, he told her to take the advice of the doctor. "Maybe," he said, "the man knows something of what he's talking about."

"That man?" she said. "If he thinks this is anything but a new mole, that shows just how much he knows. Nothing."

What Dr. Roberts told everyone privately, was that he was sure it was a form of cancer, and if he had to guess, a particularly virulent one. He said if she did not get it treated right away, it would definitely become a problem.

Harold and Dr. Roberts tried to come up with a plan to spring this information on her. Harold brought Dr. Roberts over to their house on a night when he knew Cheryl was sober. The idea was to explain the procedure for testing the cancer, but to do it in such a way that she thought it was her idea.

Unfortunately, the plan never even got off the ground. Because once Cheryl came home, she smelled out what they were doing.

She kicked Dr. Roberts out. And she went to sleep that night sure that everyone around her was an utter moron and that she would eventually be proven the superior intellect. She was sure that her strong upbringing, her will, and her spirit were enough.

She for sure did not have cancer, she thought.

Except she was wrong.

The unfortunate thing is that it took her health deteriorating quite a lot for her to realize she needed help. Dr. Roberts, being a good doctor, was of course there for her when she asked for it.

By then, however, the cancer had spread. It was getting into her lymph nodes, and it was moving fast.

But she, of course, found a way to spin it. By her reckoning, the problem was that when everyone had told her the first time it was cancer, they were wrong at that particular point in time. At that point, it was just a mole. It became cancer later, which was when she noticed that it had changed.

"I just knew," she said, usually nodding her head slowly. "There was one day I woke up, I said, there it is, Cheryl. It's changed into something else entirely."

Anyway, the end of the story is a happy one. The cancer went into remission, because she finally owned up and got the growth looked at by someone who knew what they were doing.

But what is the point of this story exactly?

The point of this story was to remind you that we cannot always pull things off on our own, and we are not always the smartest person in the room. Sometimes we encounter a situation where we do not know how best to handle it, no matter what our ego tells us. And when that happens, our best bet is to turn to someone who, yes, has superior knowledge.

This should not make us feel emasculated, or whatever the feminine version of that is. If we are having trouble losing weight, for example, or have issues with blood sugar, and we would benefit from a dietitian—why not use one?

These men and women did their due diligence, got their credentials; they have practiced their craft, and they know how to help. If you can afford one, and you are having some issues, then why not give them a shot?

It is certainly better than letting your health suffer because you were too proud to ask for a leg up.

But, yes, they are expensive. *And oftentimes, it is nonetheless true that we are capable of doing things on our own.* In fact, just as often as we refuse to get help when we need it, we are guilty of underestimating our true potential.

So, if for whatever reason, we decide to come up with meal plans on our own, how exactly do we do this?

Creating a Personalized Meal Plan

While it remains true that getting a dietitian to create your meal plan is the best option, as we discussed, it is often not the most practical. If that is the case, we need to get all our ducks in a row with regards to doing it ourselves.

And it is with that in mind that we have a few steps here which we should consider when embarking on this journey of ours (Beth, 2019).

The first you will need to think about is your schedule. Are you home often? If you are, when are you most/least busy? How often do you go to the grocery store? How often do you go out for food, or order in?

These answers will help give you an idea of which meals you should be planning for. Because through these answers, you will have a concrete timetable not just for when you can cook, but when you will have the energy to do so.

Essentially, what you want to do is figure out, on a calendar, when you will have openings to sit down and cook your meals for the week. This might only be one day, or something you have to do in pieces throughout.

The real pro-tip here is to start small and work your way up. Do one recipe for the first week, then add more as you get more comfortable. Eventually, you will know just how many meals you can make per week, sit at your comfort level and Bob's your uncle.

Next up is, of course, choosing your recipes. This is a hard one, in terms of figuring out where to begin. Not only are there gazillions of recipes out there online, but even more in all those recipe books that people buy and never use. So, how do you find a place to get your footing in this world of endless recipes?

Well, the first thing is that every one of us has different preferences as far as how long we like to cook, and how detailed, say, we like cooking to be. Myself, I do not like to cook for long periods of time, and I certainly do not like complicated recipes. Simple, short and easy ones are my favorite, so I choose recipes which fit that mold.

But maybe you are home all day and like to get other things done while cooking. You can always use a slow cooker and do housework, or put something in the oven, even. This is a great method because not only does it allow you to multitask, but it also allows you to make larger batches of things, which means having plenty of leftovers.

You should also figure out what sorts of things you store in your pantry. Do you have lots of beans, spices? Boxes of pasta? Whatever you tend to keep in your home can be a potential ingredient, and can help you determine what kinds of recipes you should be gravitating toward.

Additionally, there are all sorts of sales and seasonal things happening at the grocery store, which, if you stay on top of, can help inform what you will be making during any particular week. You can find most of these sales online, but there are apps too, like Flipp, which shows you what is on sale at stores nearby.

The pro-tip here is that the longer you do this, the more you will discover which recipes you have a preference for. And once you get there, you will have a much easier time coming up with what to make every week.

Now that we have a schedule and some recipes in mind, we can start putting those two things together. By this, I mean that we can take the recipes we have chosen and figure out when we are going to make them.

One thing we might think about though is that simply making recipes on this or that day might turn out to be a tad boring. Sometimes, as with many things in life, it helps to add a bit of a theme into the mix and see what comes out the other side.

For example: I enjoy the NFL a lot. And the Super Bowl is often a big day for me. But while having friends over and watching the game is great on its own, I like to spice things up a bit by making the whole day themed around which team I want to win.

For this reason, I started a tradition: Whichever team I want to win, for the whole day I only listen to bands from that city, and the food I make has to be one that city is known for. So, for example, if the Patriots are your team that year, then you might make clam chowder. Or if it is the Eagles, maybe you make some Philly cheesesteaks.

And honestly, it has become a tradition I look forward to every year. And meal planning can be similarly fun!

So you can, say, go Meatless Monday, or Taco Tuesday. You can have a pasta night, or a pizza night. You can even do an Around The World, global food day, just to give yourself the opportunity to try some new thing.

It might not be essential, and certainly you can do without it. But there is no doubt that it for sure makes cooking more fun, particularly if you know you are having guests over at some point.

Next up, we are going to talk about grocery lists. Which, I know, sucks. And is probably the reason most of us prefer takeout in the first place. But making a grocery list does a lot of the heavy lifting when it comes to meal planning, and is, honestly, way simpler than it sounds.

Basically, how you want to start here is by looking over all of your recipes and laying out the ingredients you will need. I know, duh. But you would be surprised by how many people skip this step!

A lot of people, in fact, just go to the grocery store, grab whatever catches their eye, and then go home. It is often when they are in their kitchen, unloading the groceries, that they realize how many things they forgot. Which, if you are anything like me, leads to this thought process:

"If I forgot X thing, then I can't make X recipe. Which I was going to eat tonight. But now I can't. So, it looks like I'll have to order takeout..."

And then the process starts all over again, spending money on things I do not need to spend money on, and on, and on. It is best to just make the dang list, stick to it, and not wind up on that treadmill of eating things you would be better off staying away from.

Now, since our focus here is on glucose, that means creating a grocery list and determining which recipes we are going to use is going to revolve around the glycemic index. Basically, we want to look at which foods are best for us, in the sense that they will help us reach our glycemic goals, if you will, and then work around that.

Since, in this scenario, we are not using a dietitian to help us make a glucose-centric meal plan, we will have to use our own eyes and brains to come up with this recipe and grocery list. This really is a simple matter of checking the ingredients in this or that recipe against the glycemic index, and seeing if maybe something needs to be subbed out, or if the meal needs to be replaced altogether.

Now, I know some of you have noticed that, in the last chapter, we already went over some specific meals which we can eat while on this diet. Which is great! But obviously some people will not enjoy those foods, or have allergies, or maybe even be vegetarian or vegan. That means putting in a bit of extra work with regards to making this plan—which is totally fine. But if and when that happens, the glycemic index is going to be our friend.

Either way, being able to throw together a meal plan that is not one-size-fits-all and can meet your needs and preferences is a good skill to have.

And speaking of good skills to have…

Reading Labels: More Important Than You Might Think!

Look, the fact of the matter is that most of us have no idea how to read nutrition labels. But this is maybe one of the more important skills out there, because what we eat is, obviously, one of the main things that leads to us being healthy or not.

We should know what we are eating, should we not? And so, with that in mind, here are some of the basics with regard to reading nutrition labels, with a specific eye toward glucose (Diabetes Care, 2022).

The ingredients list is, clearly, the part of the label which lists off what is in the food you are buying. Ingredients are listed in order of weight, so that the ingredient listed first takes up the highest percentage of the total weight of the thing, and the final ingredient listed takes up the least.

For glucose diets, we are looking at where sugar falls on this list, before anything else. If it is right near the top, then we should stay away from it. If it is somewhere near the bottom, there is a chance we may be in the clear.

Once you have done that, and you know whether or not this item contains sugar, it is time to look at the nutritional information. Here is where you will learn which kind of sugar, and how much of it, is present in this item. Also, since sugar is a carbohydrate, you are looking specifically for the word "carbohydrate" on that list.

Now, sugar, as we know, can be present in a whole bunch of different forms. So, when we look at an ingredients list, we might see words like "cane juice," "corn syrup," "dextrose," "fructose," "glucose," "honey," "lactose," "maltose," "molasses," or "sucrose". All of this means the same thing: There is sugar in this item.

As for the "daily value" percentage listed in the nutritional information, remember that a percentage of 15% or higher means there is a lot of sugar in the item (Diabetes Care, 2022). So do your best to stay away from those if you want the diet to be successful.

All in all, reading labels is a simple but essential skill when it comes to eating healthy. And since the labels make it quite clear how much sugar is present in any particular item, it is really easy to figure out whether or not the item you are interested in fits into your health plans.

And that, if you are doing it yourself, means deciding whether or not to add it to your meal plan.

***

So, what's the takeaway here?

Well, we know that when we can seek professional help, it is wise to do so. Thinking we have the same capabilities as a professional is just ridiculous and could result in us doing something that is not, as it turns out, good for us.

But, of course, professional help is expensive. So, if that means that getting help is impossible, there are shortcuts we can learn and tips that will help us get close to our goals. That might mean having to put in some extra time, but that is the tradeoff we make.

The problem, of course, is that whether we are using a dietitian or making our own meal plan, making these changes stick is a real challenge. This is, obviously, the source of the term "yo-yo dieting," where we pick up a diet, put it down, and do it all over again, time after time.

So how do we stay motivated? How do we stay on track?

There's only one way to find out. Let's turn the page!

Chapter 6:

Embracing Glucose Revolution

Hacks for Long-Term Success

With all of this behind us now, with information both theoretical and practical at our disposal, there remains one stubborn question we have not yet answered: What are we supposed to do about that pesky thing "motivation?"

This is not just some idle question either. Motivation is maybe the biggest killer when we try to make a change in our life. Exercise is maybe the most notorious for this, where getting ourselves to commit to the first day is maybe the hardest part; but if we drop our routine for even a single day, the likelihood that we will drop exercise altogether increases like crazy.

What can we do, then, to make sure we stay motivated? Are there tips and tricks we can use to keep ourselves on track?

As it turns out: yes. Very much so.

Powerful Hacks for Lifelong Glucose Control: The Keys to Long-Term Success

Cognitive-behavioral therapy is, appropriately, a type of therapy which tries to change the way you think about things, in order to change your behavior. Up until mindfulness replaced it as the favored technique in recent years, it was therapists' go-to in terms of helping people deal with various mental health problems, but especially depression and anxiety.

One of the tools of this type of therapy is known as "cognitive restructuring." This is basically where you notice the types of thoughts you have, and specifically what triggers those thoughts. Once you figure out where your, say, happy or sad thoughts come from, then the goal is to reframe them (Tigar, 2022).

Let's try an example. Say we have a goal to eat more vegetables and less, I dunno, pizza. At some point we will get a craving for pizza, that is unavoidable. At some point too, we will cave to the craving for pizza, order it, and probably eat too much of it.

The realistic response to this event is to recognize that we are only human, that we of course have temptations that we will yield to, and that while we enjoyed that pizza, we will look forward to a day of healthy eating the next day.

The problem is that for many of us, this event—ordering and eating pizza—is a sign of our own uselessness. Instead of recognizing our own ambiguity, we say, "Well, I guess I am incapable of sticking to this plan for healthy eating. So, I might as well just throw the whole thing out the window and go back to eating crap".

This "all or nothing" attitude is when we fall off the tracks, in other words. Which means that, in order to stick with a plan, whatever that plan is, we need to identify: if we are prone to that sort of thinking; what triggers that type of thinking in us; how we can reframe that thinking into something more positive and healthy (Tigar, 2022).

Obviously, this is no walk in the park. In fact, often it takes years to get this right. But even if we are trying to implement something like the glucose diet, there are going to be times when we buy a bag of Fuzzy Peaches and eat the whole thing while watching some equally-sugary movie in the theater. And for that to not derail us completely, means not succumbing to the kind of thinking that says, "If I can't do this all the time, I can't do this ever, so I might as well quit."

Next up, you need to create a clear, tangible goal that gets you excited. What do I mean by this?

This actually comes in part from the world of narrative. A story, in its essence, is when someone wants something, but encounters obstacles along the way. But the thing they want, the goal, has to be something that is "clear," meaning you can say what it is out loud, and in a way that is not confusing or ambiguous.

Consider *Raiders Of The Lost Ark*. What does Indiana Jones want? The Ark of the Covenant. The movie, the story, revolves around his attempts at getting the Ark before the Nazis do.

Another example might be *Avengers: Infinity War*, where the story revolved around the characters trying to stop Thanos from getting the Infinity Stones.

And these are just the pop culture phenomenon versions of this. Murder mysteries revolve around questions like, "Who was the killer?" Horror movies revolve around attempts at destroying a monster. In murder mysteries, the story is over when the murder is solved. In horror stories, the story is over when the monster is destroyed (or all the other characters are).

This works for us in part because of its simplicity. We know what the characters have to do; we know, given the genre, roughly what they will do to get it, and we know when to expect the story to be over.

With diet, the same principles apply. We have a clear, tangible goal—say, eating a certain number of planned meals per week—and we feel accomplishment, and therefore motivation, when we achieve those goals.

But another secret to this is to make your goal exciting. What do I mean here? Well, maybe you are an artistic person who gets excited by visual images. Why not find visuals which embody your vision of success? Merely having them around might be enough to keep you motivated (Tigar, 2022).

Whatever you choose, make sure it is based on something that makes you feel like you want to push yourself through the rough patches—because, rest assured, there will be those. So, whether you are visual or auditory, or whatever else, something that gives you that sense of joy and motivation is going to be one of the keys to your success.

Another thing to think about too, with regard to goals, is whether it would be better to pare them down to micro-goals.

The fact of the matter is that we can easily get overwhelmed by how distant our goals might seem, particularly if they are of a lofty nature. Maybe we want to lose a certain amount of weight, or eat healthy a certain number of cumulative days over the course of a month. Breaking down, say, the 30 pounds we want to lose into five-to-ten pound chunks can help give us that dopamine rush from when we know we have accomplished something, but more often than we would by simply focusing on the big goal. This way, we are way more likely to stay motivated (Tigar, 2022).

Related to cognitive reframing too is the idea that we should not just think about what our goals are, but why we want to achieve them (Tigar, 2022). Goals that come from a place of negativity are more likely to cause stress, which means we will associate them with that emotion more and more over time, which means we will be less likely to continue pursuing them.

But beyond that, we want to make sure that our intentions are good. If we want to lose weight but want to do it because we think it will finally make someone love us, then we need to regroup and rethink what our priorities are. Wanting to lose weight for health reasons, meanwhile, is a noble and sensible reason for pursuing that goal, provided it is non-pathological and does not come from, say, an eating disorder.

Another thing to think of too is the buddy system. We are all familiar with this one: Essentially, we make our intentions known to someone who can help keep us honest. Maybe this is someone who has similar goals to us, or a loved one who wants to help us reach ours. Either way, having someone to keep you on track is a good idea, provided you do not saddle someone else with the burden of your problems (Tigar, 2022).

This last part is an important one. Throughout my own life, I have known tons of people who have brought other people into their problems, ostensibly to get help, but really just to make their problem someone else's. This tactic has, I would guess, a 0% success rate, and should be avoided at all costs.

It is also super mean. So do not do this.

What you can do also is make a list of what the benefits of your goal will, or might, be. So, if you are going on the glucose diet, you could make a list of things like: losing weight; gaining mental clarity; having more energy throughout the day. Or whatever it is about this diet that makes you interested in implementing it (Tigar, 2022).

In doing so, you will be reminding yourself that what you are doing is not just for the hell of it. You have reasons for doing this, and reasons that will be to your benefit. When reaching the goals gets hard, then, you have all these nice reasons laying around to remind of what accomplishing your goals will hopefully look like.

And finally: Do not be afraid of acknowledging your wins!

Depending on who you are as a person, this may be easy, or it may be challenging. Certainly, I see both around me all the time. Social media in particular is filled with people celebrating even the smallest victories; but I know lots of people in person who think saying they accomplished something is somehow bad form.

The best way to do this, for my money, is somewhere in between. We should be sensible enough to realize that when we do accomplish something, it really is worth celebrating. We are not being arrogant, or indulging in hubris, by admitting that we did something cool. We are acknowledging the facts of the matter, which means we are being realistic.

Now, what you may have noticed here is that our mental state has a significant impact on our ability to meet our goals.

So, what happens if we zoom in a little on this? What else can we learn about mental states, how they affect us, and which mental states we should be trying to enter into to accomplish our goals?

Mastering Your Mindset: Unleashing the Force Behind Long-Term Glucose Success

One thing we can look into is whether we have a "fixed" mindset, or a "growth" mindset, i.e., whether we think that things are the way they are and can never change, or that by applying pressure to things, working hard and adapting, we can create positive, incremental changes in our lives (Scudamore, 2017).

I know, I know. This sounds like it is from some bad self-help book. But there really is some wisdom to this.

For example, I used to have a friend who was living the kind of life he had always hoped he would not. He was working a job he did not like, living in an apartment he hated, and, frankly, was miserable every second of the day.

Every year there would come a time when he would say he was going to apply to college. He would get all jazzed about it, collect information from those of us who had been already, and start to make plans to put this in action. But every year, the same thought would derail him: "What's the point? Nothing is going to get any better. I am not going to get in. I am going to be stuck here for the rest of my life. Why would I even bother trying to make things change when they won't?"

You can imagine how this went for him. His stresses piled up, he became more and more down on himself—until, eventually, something had to change.

"I decided one day that I wasn't going to think like that anymore," he said. "I decided that I'd been wrong, and that I could change my life if I wanted. At the very least, I owed it to myself to try."

What happened then, was he got his application together, got into college, graduated a year early, and now works his dream job at a small press publisher in Chicago. In other words, once he decided to change the way he thought about his life, he was able to actually change his life.

And you can do this too!

Whether you are starting the glucose diet because you are unhappy with your weight, want to improve focus, whatever it is, recognizing that you have the ability to change is going to get you the results you want. And, what's more, recognizing that you have the ability to take control of your life and get where you want is one the keys to staying motivated.

If you keep telling yourself that you cannot succeed, then you will give up. If you tell yourself that you can, and you will, then the world will be your oyster.

Another thing you can do, which is maybe the hardest of all, is to stop fearing failure and embrace it.

As I said, this is maybe the hardest to do. But consider some of the most successful people in history, particularly in athletics. What they were was prolific, meaning they tried again and again, and failed the vast majority of the time.

Consider the batter with the best batting average in baseball. That would be Ty Cobb, with a batting average of something like 0.366 (ESPN, 2023). Because of how batting averages are calculated, that means he hit the ball in only a third of his at-bats. And he is still the greatest of all time, batting-wise.

Accomplishing something, and in particular being successful at something, does not mean hitting a home run every time you get up to bat. Being a human being means that the vast majority of what you do will not pan out. And that sucks! Believe me, I know it does. But that is still the best we have got, and that is what we have to live with.

Embracing this fact is one of the ways you will properly ensure your success. Being afraid means not getting up to bat at all and getting a zero on the scorecard. Success means getting up and failing, still, two-thirds of the time.

Translating this into practical terms for us, then: If we want to eat well, using the glycemic index as our guide, and exercise, and do everything else suggested in this book, in order to achieve maximum good health—we have to accept that there are still going to be times when we utterly flub it. As we talked about earlier, reframing these failures is a big part of making sure they do not sink you. But that means not being scared to fail, recognizing failure as a part of life, and keeping your mind set on the big picture.

And ultimately, that leads us to our final point with regards to mindset: staying positive.

There are some people out there for whom staying positive is the easiest thing in the world. If you are one of these people, then congratulations. I myself have encountered these people in the wild and am often super confused as to how they manage to pull such a thing off.

For me, positivity has never come easy. It is a real uphill battle to try and see the bright side in things, not to "catastrophize," as the kids are calling it, and not just assume that the worst thing ever is right around the corner.

But the thing is, being positive does not have to mean being gullible. It does not mean you have to believe that literally everything is sunshine and rainbows, or to make yourself, effectively, into an easy mark. It just means recognizing the world for what it is: ambiguous. Neither all bad nor all good. Requiring both, on some level, to continue on. And requiring that you accept this in order to succeed in it.

Really, this is just being realistic. Because hard work does reward you eventually, if sometimes only in ways you did not expect. Creating a plan does make accomplishing your goals easier. And adopting healthy lifestyle choices does make you feel better and is more likely to help you live longer too.

For us, that means knowing that just because we failed one time does not mean we will fail every time. It means knowing that if we lay the groundwork, we have a solid foundation on which to build our plan for success. Not that our plan is foolproof, because even child-proof lids can be taken off by kids, often quite easily. But given enough time, and enough at-bats, we can achieve a measure of success that we could previously only dream of.

But, of course, doing so is not exactly easy. And all those obstacles you encounter along the way are sure to make you stressed out, which, as we said before, is not healthy in the absolute slightest.

What then can we do to make sure we stay level-headed and not get stressed out?

Stress Management: A Primer

Stress management is a topic that honestly could have—and does have—several books written on it. So, whatever we say here is going to be cursory at best, despite how important it is.

And why is it important? Well, since we are talking about diet and exercise, we should be mindful of the fact that many of our dietary choices, such as overeating, and eating junk, result from poor stress management. We are looking for the rush we get from food in order to make ourselves feel level.

And if we do not use food in this way, consider also that plans are often derailed when we get stressed out and decide it would be easier to go back to our old ways. The devil that we know, in a sense, is better than the one we do not.

Better managing our stress is a sure-fire way to make sure we do not fall into either of those patterns. Because if we can manage stress without using food, then we will not be tempted into terrible eating habits. And if we can manage the stress that naturally comes with lifestyle changes and encountering a challenging obstacle, then we will not revert back to our old, unhealthy ways.

But how exactly do we manage stress?

Maybe one of the best things you can do is to encounter stress as a problem-solver. Problem-solving is built into our psyches. That is why we make tools, and how we were able to build cities, cure disease and send people up into space. Human beings encounter problems, and we solve them. (Likely every other animal in the world does this too, but you get the point.)

Stress comes as a result of running into something that thwarts our plans or makes them more difficult. This means we have found an obstacle. But instead of figuring out how to get around it, we get stressed, which often makes us more likely to abandon our plans.

Coming at obstacles like a problem-solver means finding a way around the stressor. For example, maybe we are trying to eat better but Christmas is coming up. We know we have a tendency to eat sugary junk over Christmas, and we really do not want to.

One response would be to give in to excessive worry. In that scenario, we become stressed, wondering how in the hell we are ever going to get through the holidays. We might see this as so insurmountable that we decide to just throw in the towel and have a whole week of white wine, candy canes, and white bread.

Another response though, would be to come up with a plan. We could recognize that it is fine to have sugary junk some of the time, that it is the holidays, and the holidays are a safe time when things like this happen. Or we could figure out how to meditate, maybe use mindfulness techniques to get through our desire to rip off the band-aid and go hog wild with carbs.

Whatever you decide to do, coming up with a plan means solving the problem, means eliminating the stress. Maybe not completely, but enough to make the stress less, well, stressful.

And if you do that, then you are ensuring your chances of success have just gone up.

You also might want to try being more organized. I know, it sounds like I am attacking you. But I am not!

This totally grows out of the same notion as being stressed. When we are not organized, when we allow our days to be chaotic, we are more prone to give into impulse. When our impulses control us, then we are in trouble. But what happens when *we* control our impulses? Well, then it is trouble that is in trouble.

Being organized in this sense means that we have meal plans, we have a fridge that is stocked, we have a plan for what to do if and when we get the urge to go hog wild. All of our ducks are in a row, so to speak, which leaves us with way less opportunity to start fretting about what we are going to do for, say, dinner, before we decide to just use Uber Eats to drop off a tub of ice cream.

Reducing the chaos in our life will also make us worry less in general. Maybe we need to clean our apartment or do our laundry. Maybe we need to organize our bookshelves. Whatever it is, if something in our life is chaotic, it causes us stress. And when we are stressed, we start to make silly mistakes.

But sometimes that is not realistic, right? Sometimes things are busy and hectic, there is no time to keep the fridge stocked, we are not reaching our goals… In those scenarios, it can feel like we are going to be stressed and there is nothing we can do about it.

Or is there?

Before we decide that the pressure is too much and we are just going to throw in the towel, remember that dealing with these types of situations can be as simple as just taking a few minutes for yourself. Or even just a single minute! Go into your bedroom, lay down, turn off the lights. Close your eyes. You can even time yourself. But having a whole minute to collect yourself, getting your thoughts in order, and then going back out to face the day, can really make all the difference in the world.

We can take stock of our accomplishments so far, if we have been keeping track of them. (And we should be.) We can remember that we are only human, and life is challenging by nature. And when we have found a good center, calmed ourselves and made peace with our circumstances, we can go back out into the world to face whatever problem we have with a fresh pair of eyes, and a renewed vigor for success.

In short, any change we try to implement is going to be stressful. But if we think of stressors as problems that need to be solved, maintain a high degree of preparedness and organization, and take a minute to find perspective and keep ourselves calm, we can kick that stress straight in the teeth and send it packing.

Of course, that is not all. Maybe we draw strength from strong social connections, or strength from the arts and music. Maybe there is a movie that helps us manage our stress better, or a sport we like to play casually.

Whatever it is, we all have our ways of dealing with stress. So long as it is healthy, and so long as it works, then I say go for it. Accomplishing your goals is hard, and if it helps, then it helps.

Just remember to keep your eye on the big picture and I know you will be fine.

***

Which leaves us where?

Well, staying motivated can be a challenging task. But what connects all that we have discussed, is that motivation is something that happens in your mind. It requires a way of seeing the world, and of looking at problems, that allows you to face adversity and conquer the things that are holding you back.

You are more than capable of achieving that mindset. I know it, because we all are.

Which leaves us with only a few more words left. So, as we get ready to part ways, let's go on one more short little journey together.

It's time to wrap this whole thing up. We're off to the conclusion.

Conclusion

What, at the end of the day, is the glucose revolution?

And where should we begin, except right back at the beginning?

After that day at the emu farm, I started to wonder if our body wasn't best looked at holistically. Everything from our diet to how we exercise and how often, how we handle stress—everything seems connected. Every choice we make leaves some kind of an imprint on our bodies, for which we deal with the consequences later.

Blood sugar, it seems, is an indicator of how healthy we are, and how healthy we feel. Every one of these actions, diet and exercise and everything else, has an impact on our blood sugar, which in turn, makes us feel everything from focused and energized, to dizzy and weak.

Caring for our blood sugar, in other words, is identical to caring for ourselves, body and mind.

Throughout the course of this book, we have covered a whole host of ways we can take care of our blood sugar. We know now that food is the primary way to do this, and we looked over the glycemic index as a way to measure the healthiness of the food we eat. We went over how exercise balances our blood sugar out over time, even if it spikes it temporarily. And, of course, we covered how stress can do horrible things to our blood sugar and should be kept to a minimum, when possible.

In addition, we went over glucose monitors and how they are most probably useless for the majority of us, and how dietitians are awesome but expensive. As a result, by now we should know how to make a meal plan, how to keep ourselves organized, and how to know if our blood sugar has gone out of whack simply by studying our symptoms.

But mostly, I think, we know now that blood sugar is more than just an issue for people with diabetes. It is something that affects us all, and through it we can unlock the secrets of our success.

***

I said earlier I do not know what happened to Shana Rey after she left my school. And that is partly true: There is a whole period of her life that is a mystery to me, probably fifteen or so years.

But I did actually run into her one more time. Just a few years ago.

I was in a local grocery store by myself, shopping through the vegetable aisle. I practice what I preach: I had a grocery cart filled with whole grains, fruit, and an assortment of vegetables. And it was just as I picked up a cabbage to inspect, that I saw her come around the corner.

It is weird seeing someone you knew as a child, but who is now an adult. Especially someone with whom you share only one memory, significant though it is. For a second, I was not even sure it was her. But my leering must have caught her attention, because she snuck a glance over at me.

And recognized me right away.

We did not spend that much time talking, to be honest. We mentioned how weird it was to see each other, how much time had passed, that sort of thing. We talked about the grocery store, the weather... Although never, I see now, about what life had been like since we had seen each other last. Nothing about work, love—just small talk.

I did manage to bring up that incident at the farm though. And it was odd, but she did not seem to remember at first. Her eyes glazed over and she thought about it for a moment, before the memory flickered across her eyes and she laughed.

"I haven't thought about that in years," she said. "Honestly, it's not the only time I've had something like that happen to me. It took a while before I got a handle on my diabetes."

"But you do now? Have a handle on it, I mean?"

She looked at me cock-eyed and said, "Well, I wouldn't be here if I didn't, would I?"

I had to laugh at that. But what I wanted to tell her was how significant that moment on the farm had been for me. Because of it I had learned a lot about health, especially how blood sugar relates to that.

But that would have seemed forced. So, all I said was, "How do you do it?"

I saw she knew what I meant. I wanted to know how she managed to put so much thought and effort into keeping herself healthy. Especially when she had a death machine dangling over her head.

This time, it was her turn to laugh. And she said, "It's for my health, ain't it? What else am I supposed to do?"

She was right, of course. Soon after that, she left. And that was the last time I had seen her, and likely the last time I ever would.

But there is such a pearl of wisdom in that interaction with her, that I would like more than anything to leave with it in mind.

If she slips in terms of taking care of herself, the consequences could be severe and immediate. For people without diabetes, if they slip occasionally, they will probably be fine. It is many slips over long periods of time that add up for them.

So maybe it is not fair to compare people with diabetes to those without. But nonetheless, she recognizes that since it is her health on the line, of course she should put the time in to make sure she stays healthy. Not doing so means getting sick, or worse.

And who wants that?

It really is a matter of priority. Saying that our minds and bodies matter means admitting that we should take care of them. And taking care of them means not just eating right, but exercising, learning how to practice cognitive reframing, sleeping well—all things, as we have seen, that impact our blood glucose.

Shana knows full well that her health matters, because she has seen, too many times, what happens when she does not pay attention. The lesson for us then is not that what happens to her could happen to us; it is instead that what we put into our bodies, and how we treat them, impacts a whole slew of other things downwind from food and exercise.

Which is what, I think, separates this book from fad diet books. I hope by now you will agree with me, but as we said before, there are so many different versions of "cure-all" diets out there, so much confusing information, so much, frankly, quackery. Sifting through all that would require more time than any of us have on-hand, ever.

What I am saying here is much simpler than what is in any of those other books: Blood sugar is a measure of the healthiness of the food you eat, how much exercise you get, and where your mental health is at. Eating well, exercising, and staying sane, are all things any reasonable person would recommend.

And hopefully, if I have done my job right, you now have the tools to pull that off.

***

Which is where we part, Dear Reader. We have been like two passengers on a plane, sitting next to one another, trying to arrive at the same destination. It is somewhere I have been before, and somewhere, I think, you are only just getting to now.

But it is somewhere you are getting to, nonetheless.

Just remember: When you step off that ramp, you are landing on new ground. The sun will be warm. The people will be friendly. There will be a thousand sights to see, and the nights will be like an endless party.

If you can stay here, you will find peace. But staying here means keeping a good head on your shoulders.

And how do you do that? It is just a matter of staying motivated. Because when you lose your motivation, you have to get back on the plane and start again. You will always be welcome back, of course. But it is always better to stay.

Because the sun really is shining all the time here. You will feel warm and happy, you will get to go for long walks on the beach, and you will appear with a confidence you never thought you had.

You will have the confidence of someone who has seen their goals, identified them, and gone for them. Someone who does not get bogged down by missed attempts or obstacles. The kind of person who can see the importance of healthy living, and who is willing to grind it out to get there.

That is the destination you have arrived at. And with a lot of hard work and perseverance, you can, without a doubt, stay here for as long as you want.

Welcome to the glucose revolution.

Congratulations on reaching the end of Glucose Revolution Hacks!

I hope you feel empowered with new knowledge and tools to take control of your glucose levels and health.

As a thank you for joining me on this journey, I have a special gift for you - a 7-day meal plan to kickstart your new, healthier lifestyle! This plan includes nourishing breakfasts, lunches, and dinners with complete recipes, ingredients, instructions, nutritional information, and benefits.

Simply scan the QR code to download your free gift.

I carefully designed these recipes to help regulate blood sugar and make healthy eating enjoyable. You deserve delicious food that nourishes your body! Follow this meal plan to ease into better habits with less stress. You've taken the first step by reading this book - now put that knowledge into action.

I believe in you! Stay positive, be patient with yourself, and let healthy eating become a celebration. This is the beginning of a happier, healthier you!

I hope you enjoyed Glucose Revolution Hacks and found it helpful on your health journey.

If so, I would be incredibly grateful if you would take a moment to leave a review, sharing your thoughts about the book. Your feedback will mean a lot, as it will help other readers who are looking to improve their glucose levels and overall wellbeing decide if this book is for them.

Your review will also support me in creating more content that empowers people to take control of their health. Whether you have a brief comment or an in-depth review to share, please know that I greatly appreciate you taking the time. It is readers like you and your support that keep me motivated to continue providing helpful information.

Thank you again for reading Glucose Revolution Hacks! I hope it sparked positive changes in your life.

Wishing you all the best,

Olivia Rivers

References

Ajmera, R. (2023, March 3). *Glycemic index: What it is and how to use it.* Healthline. https://www.healthline.com/nutrition/glycemic-index#low-glycemic-diet.

Beth. (2019, December 15). *Meal planning 101 - How to make a custom meal plan.* Budget Bytes www.budgetbytes.com/meal-planning-101-how-to-make-a-meal-plan-that-works-for-you/.

Centers for Disease Control and Prevention (CDC). (2021, January 20). *Low blood sugar (hypoglycemia).* Centers for Disease Control and Prevention. www.cdc.gov/diabetes/basics/low-blood-sugar.html.

Chalicha, E. (2021, August 5). *7-Day low glycemic diet plan: Keep your blood sugar steady with these meals.* BetterMe Blog. betterme.world/articles/7-day-low-glycemic-diet-plan/.

Cleveland Clinic. (2020, February 11). *Hyperglycemia signs, treatment & prevention.* Cleveland Clinic. my.clevelandclinic.org/health/diseases/9815-hyperglycemia-high-blood-sugar.

College of Dietitians of Alberta (n.d.). *What do dietitians do?* College of Dietitians of Alberta. collegeofdietitians.ab.ca/public/what-do-dietitians-do/.

Crider, C. (2023, July 7). *Hypoglycemia and weight loss: What you should know.* Healthline. www.healthline.com/health/hypoglycemia-and-weight-loss#takeaway. Accessed 21 Aug. 2023.

Cronkleton, E. (2019, July 12). *Warmup exercises: 6 ways to get warmed up before a workout.* Healthline. www.healthline.com/health/fitness-exercise/warm-up-exercises#bottom-line.

Diabetes Care. (2018, September 7). *Exercise plan for diabetes - daily, weekly, monthly* Diabetes Care Community. www.diabetescarecommunity.ca/diet-and-fitness-articles/physical-activity-articles/exercise-planning/exercise-plan-diabetes/. Accessed 21 Aug. 2023.

Diabetes Care. (2022, December 20). *Understanding sugar content on food labels.* Diabetes Care Community. www.diabetescarecommunity.ca/diet-and-fitness-articles/understanding-sugar-content-on-food-labels/. Accessed 21 Aug. 2023.

Edwards, S. (2016). *Sugar and the brain.* Harvard Medical School. hms.harvard.edu/news-events/publications-archive/brain/sugar-brain.

ESPN. (2023). *MLB career batting leaders.* ESPN. https://www.espn.com/mlb/history/leaders

Johnson, E. (2022). *8 ways balancing your blood sugar can improve your health.* Veri. www.veri.co/learn/7-benefits-of-stable-blood-sugar.

Long, T. (2020). *Regulation of Blood Glucose.* ATrain Education. www.atrainceu.com/content/4-regulation-blood-glucose.

National Institute of Diabetes and Digestive and Kidney Diseases. (2019). *Preventing type 2 diabetes.* National Institute of Diabetes and Digestive and Kidney Diseases. www.niddk.nih.gov/health-information/diabetes/overview/preventing-type-2-diabetes.

National Institute of Diabetes and Digestive and Kidney Diseases. (2023). *Continuous glucose monitoring*. National Institute of Diabetes and Digestive and Kidney Diseases. www.niddk.nih.gov/health-information/diabetes/overview/managing-diabetes/continuous-glucose-monitoring#:~:text=A%20continuous%20glucose%20monitor%20(CGM. Accessed 14 Aug. 2023.

Pacheco, D. (2020, December 4). *Sleep & glucose: How blood sugar can affect rest*. Sleep Foundation. www.sleepfoundation.org/physical-health/sleep-and-blood-glucose-levels.

Porterfield, C. *Just 28% of Americans are exercising enough, CDC says—and it's even lower in some regions*. Forbes. www.forbes.com/sites/carlieporterfield/2023/01/26/just-28-of-americans-are-exercising-enough-cdc-says-and-its-even-lower-in-some-regions/?sh=79d9ef682b96. Accessed 21 Aug. 2023.

Sass, C. (2015, January 30). *6 things you should know about working with a nutritionist*. Health.com. www.health.com/celebrities/6-things-you-should-know-about-working-with-a-nutritionist-dietitian.

Scudamore, B. (2017, August 23). *7 mindsets of highly successful (and happy) people*. Forbes. www.forbes.com/sites/brianscudamore/2017/08/23/7-mindsets-of-highly-successful-and-happy-people/?sh=6350e9d823ed. Accessed 21 Aug. 2023.

Sharma, K., et al. (2022, September 13). *Stress-induced diabetes: a review*. Cureus, vol. 14, no. 9. https://doi.org/10.7759/cureus.29142.

Shmerling, R. (2021, June 11). *Is blood sugar monitoring without diabetes worthwhile?* Harvard Health. www.health.harvard.edu/blog/is-blood-sugar-monitoring-without-diabetes-worthwhile-202106112473.

Supersapiens. (2022, May 30). *How your glucose levels impact focus.* Supersapiens. blog.supersapiens.com/how-glucose-levels-impact-focus/. Accessed 21 Aug. 2023.

Team Nutrisense. (2023, April 11). *Exercise & glucose: Why fitness impacts your glucose levels.* Team Nutrisense. www.nutrisense.io/blog/exercise-blood-glucose.

The Levels Team. (2020, June 13). *Can controlling my glucose levels give me more energy?* Levels. www.levelshealth.com/blog/can-controlling-my-glucose-levels-give-me-more-energy.

Tigar, L. (2022, November 20). *8 psychology-based tricks for staying motivated and accomplishing your goals.* Real Simple. www.realsimple.com/work-life/life-strategies/inspiration-motivation/how-to-accomplish-goals-psychologist-tips.

Walker Family Care (n.d.). *How does diabetes affect energy levels?* Walker Family Care. www.walkerfc.com/blog/how-does-diabetes-affect-energy-levels#:~:text=Because%20blood%20glucose%27s%20primary%20function.

Wright, S. and Aline Dias. (2022, July 15). *What is glucose and what does it do?* Healthline. www.healthline.com/health/glucose#typical-levels.